GW00585816

Intermittent Fasting 16/8

A Quick Start Guide For Every Age And Stage To Fight Bad Nutrition, Reduce Belly Fat, Overcome Hunger Attacks, And Discover How To Lose Weight Without Dieting.

© Copyright 2020 - All rights reserved.

The content contained within this book may not be reproduced, duplicated or transmitted without direct written permission from the author or the publisher.

Under no circumstances will any blame or legal responsibility be held against the publisher, or author, for any damages, reparation, or monetary loss due to the information contained within this book. Either directly or indirectly.

Legal Notice:

This book is copyright protected. This book is only for personal use. You cannot amend, distribute, sell, use, quote or paraphrase any part, or the content within this book, without the consent of the author or publisher.

Disclaimer Notice:

Please note the information contained within this document is for educational and entertainment purposes only. All effort has been executed to present accurate, up to date, and reliable, complete information. No warranties of any kind are declared or implied. Readers acknowledge that the author is not engaging in the rendering of legal, financial, medical or professional advice. The content within this book has been derived from various sources. Please consult a licensed professional before attempting any techniques outlined in this book.

By reading this document, the reader agrees that under no circumstances is the author responsible for any losses, direct or indirect, which are incurred as a result of the use of information contained within this document, including, but not limited to, — errors, omissions, or inaccuracies.

ISBN:

Table of Contents

Introduction

How Do You Do Intermittent Fasting?

I'm going to be talking with you about fasting and, more particularly, intermittent fasting. Now intermittent fasting is something I do. It has many different benefits, including:

- Weight loss.
- Detoxification.
- Reducing bloating.
- Improving digestion.
- And much more.

So, you've probably heard of plain old traditional fasting. I mean, it's mentioned in many things throughout history, including a lot of religious books. So, you can do that kind of fasting where you only consume water for one to three days, or you can do it where you only have one meal a day again for one to three days. You can do a juice cleanse or juice fast where you only drink fruit and vegetable juice still for one to three days. With those kinds of fasting after about three days, it becomes pretty hard on your body, and so at that point, it's no longer beneficial to your health.

Now intermittent fasting gives you all the benefits of fasting while allowing you to get enough nutrition for your system. So that's why you're able to keep it up for one to three months rather than date. Here's how it works, so we're going to fast or not consume anything except water for a certain period every day. Now don't go crazy with this. We still want a pretty decent window for eating around four to eight hours, during which time we can fit a few meals.

Personally, my eating window is between seven and eight hours. So, I'll have my first meal of breakfast at around twelve. Then three I might have lunch snack at five and dinner between seven and eight. I have a longer eating window because this is a lifestyle for me. You know it's not a temporary diet that I can only sustain for one to three months; this is long-term.

But of course, if you want to have faster results, you can shorten, you're eating window to around four hours and do that for one to three months. What this shorter eating schedule does is it allows our gut to rest a lot of us will get up at safe 7:00 in the morning, eat our first meal immediately and then continue feeding throughout the day until maybe even 10:00 p.m.

If we continue to snack after dinner, so our digestive systems never have any time to rest, it's like when you finish working out, and you're supposed to let your muscles relax and heal. But we never give that to our guts. It's like we only give it maybe eight hours a day. But when we only eat for four to eight hours a day, we're giving our gut a 16 to 20-hour rest, which improves digestion, which can reduce bloating, which will give you a flatter tummy. Now one of the best benefits of intermittent fasting is that it can balance your hormone, and it can increase your body's production of human growth hormone by 400%. Now human growth hormone isn't just for growing kids and teens; it's the primary fat-burning hormone, and it helps:

- Prevent muscle loss.
- Increases muscle strength.
- Anti-aging.
- Improve your mood.
- Cognitive function.

Another way to increase HGH, which is what week school kids are calling human growth hormone, is by doing hit workout. We've talked about when to eat, but what about what to eat when doing intermittent fasting. You're going to want to make sure you get a lot of: -

- Healthy protein.
- Fat fiber.
- Eat a lot of nutrient-dense fruit.
- Eat a lot of nutrient-dense vegetables.

So pretty much you're going to want to do the ketogenic or keto diet.

How Much Weight Can You Lose Doing Intermittent Fasting?

How much weight can you lose doing intermittent fasting? In the last five months, I've lost 70 pounds doing intermittent fasting, but the answer to the question depends on the model that you're using. I'm sure it depends on your metabolism. Of course, what you're eating so.

I'll tell you a little bit about what's worked for me and what my expectations are for myself because I've come to learn that my weight loss is very formulaic and is dependent on well what I'm eating and when I'm eating. So, I eat in a one-hour window a day, and I eat one meal in that one hour so for 23 hours I'm not eating and for one hour I am eating.

I'm eating a meal that is very low in carbohydrates; it tends to be loaded with vegetables and includes some protein. In my experience, this approach has been by far the best weight loss method I've been on save like a water fast, which jump-started my whole five-month experience. I was on 16-day water quickly in the very beginning, but aside from that, this eating in a one-hour window has been beneficial.

In my case, I can lose 10 to 15 pounds a month doing this fast, and that range is dependent on what I'm eating each day. For comparison, I lost 20 pounds in the four months before this program, and it was all low-carb, and I was losing at the rate of 4 to 5 pounds a month. So, about a pound a week and so that's just from a regular low-carb diet. I was eating very similar things, but it wasn't within that one-hour window. Now I'm losing more than twice that amount, and so my weight loss is far more rapid with the one-hour eating window.

My range is from about 10 pounds to 15 pounds a month. What I find is that I can lose closer to 15 pounds a month if my one meal a day is relatively calorie-restricted. If my meal a day is more in the 500-calorie range, then I'm going to lose closer to 15 pounds in that month. If it's more in the thousand calorie range, I'm going to drop closer to 10 pounds a month.

I mean to me that's every I don't know ten days, or so it's not a lot of meals. But at home, sometimes, if I want to incorporate something you see a lot of extra fat salmon cheese's the meals are closer to a thousand calories. I have some delicious filling meals that are 500 calories, and I'm going to post some of those 500 calorie recipes for you to give you some ideas in case you haven't thought of some of these things because you know 15 pounds a month. I mean, that's a stinking a lot of weight right. I can't even believe it; I've never lost that much weight on any diet.

Of course, the water fasting and so obviously if you need to lose weight faster may be for health reasons or some other consideration. I can quickly lose the 15 pounds if I'm doing that so as you know. You eat a thousand calories every other day, and you eat zero every other day. It's not very difficult to do a 48-hour fast right now I'm not doing it. Because I feel like a little need a little bit more daily nutrition and so, I'm going back and forth between lower-calorie meals and then the thousand calorie meals.

I'm just making sure I'm always taking a liquid vitamin and mineral supplement.

Why Does Intermittent Fasting Work?

Intermittent fasting is a simple concept that is practically defined by its name; it involves incorporating periods of fasting into your diet now. The length of time for intermittent fasting varies. But a popular time frame is 16-8, meaning that you fast for 16 hours and consume all of your calories within an eight-hour eating window. This method of timing you're eating has proven to be very useful for even stubborn metabolisms. But to appreciate why it works, we need to take a fresh look at how weight loss happens. We used to think that the calorie in calorie out model was how we lost weight.

This meant that all calories were equal, so a hundred calories of meat same 200 calories of cake, which equals 200 calories of salad. When you consumed those calories, they went into a collective bucket in your body and sat there until you needed some energy at which time the calories in the bucket were released and burned the logic was that you burn more calories. Then you consume, and weight loss happened in that model of how the body burned fat seemed logical.

It didn't seem to work. The calories in the calories out model have been the predominant way of thinking for the past 60 years, which was a period that was marked by skyrocketing obesity rates. The reason it doesn't work. Because calories are not simply dumped into a collective bucket in our bodies. Instead, they are directed into two separate storage containers and store it as either glycogen or fat. The movement into those storage containers is controlled by a hormone called insulin.

So, insulin shows up when food is coming in, and when insulin is present, food energy is being stored not released. Which is vital food energy moves in one direction at a time? It's either being saved or being released. It all depends on how much insulin is present is an easy-to-access container because it is permanently stored glucose, which is very easy for your body to burn.

But this glycogen container is small. You only have about 2,000 calories of available energy stored as glycogen fat. On the other hand, it has a lot of energy; just one pound of fat has about 3500 calories worth of energy. But that is hard to access for your body to go to the trouble of burning body fat for energy. Two things must happen; you must be running low on glycogen and have a low level of insulin in your blood.

How do you get to that state you stretch out the time between meals? In other words, you follow an intermittent fasting strategy if you are frequently eating throughout the day? You are continually refilling glycogen stores and bumping up insulin. Because there is a constant supply of glycogen, there's no need for your body to go to the trouble of converting fat into energy even if your body wanted to burn fat. It can't access it because the insulin level never drops to a point where fat can be released. When you stretch out the time between meals by practicing intermittent fasting, your body burns through some of the storage of glycogen and insulin levels drop, making that a logical choice for your body to run on now.

What Can I Eat During Intermittent Fasting?

When I do get hungry usually around the 16-hour mark after yesterday's meal or around 1:00 p.m. With this example, I've got a couple of options for what we'll call lunch even though technically it's breakfast. So, if I did not have a rocket fuel latte or a bone broth to extend the fast, I'll usually have one with this lunch bacon asparagus cooked in bacon grease kimchi and a rock a few lattes. It's relatively light, but we'll also make and keep you full for a pretty long time.

If I did have a rocket fuel latte or bone broth to extend my fast in the morning, I'd usually want more volume when breaking my fast with something like cucumbers with sauerkraut kale sautéed in mounds of coconut oil leftover shredded pork sands the sauces sautéed in coconut oil until crisp with green onions. You have got to try this meal. It's delectable and perfectly balanced then about six to eight hours after that breakfast slash lunged.

Here a couple of other options to spark your meal creativity

- Arugula tossed with olive oil.
- Balsamic topped with beef.

- Pork combo burger patties with salt pepper.
- Horseradish sauerkraut sautéed with asparagus.
- A bit of carrot cooked with lard.
- Some jicama chips.

Of course, everything is drizzled with even more oil your gut is going to love you with this one now if I'm doing a carb up with this second meal. I'll want way less fat on my plate, so we'll go with something like this grass-fed bison kimchi and some greens with a bit of avocado oil apple cider vinegar maple syrup and topped with a chopped apple and some raisins this has everything you need to stay happy and satisfied. Through your carb-up, finally, if I get hungry come nighttime, I'll spring for a keto milkshake or a delicious fat bomb.

Chapter 1

How Intermittent Fasting Works?

Intermittent fasting refers to meal planning that alternates between fasting and eating periods. The purpose is to burn physically long enough to burn body fat. Although research is currently underway and this method may not be suitable for everyone. There is evidence that, when done correctly. Intermittent fasting can:

- Reduce weight.
- Reduce blood pressure.
- Reduce cholesterol.
- Control of diabetes.
- Improve brain health.

During meals, the carbohydrates in the diet are broken down into glucose. Glucose is absorbed into the bloodstream through the intestinal wall and transported to various organs, where it is an essential source of energy. Excess glucose is stored in the form of glycogen and fat for later use in the liver and adipose tissue. When the body is in a fast state between meals, the liver converts glucose back into glucose to continue supplying energy to the body.

Usually, an inactive person takes 10-12 hours to consume glycogen stores. However, anyone who exercises can do so in a short time. Once glycogen is depleted in the liver, the body is absorbed into the tissues of the body in energy deposits. When fat is broken down into free fatty acids, they are then converted into extra metabolic fuel in the liver.

In this way, if the fasting condition lasts for a long time. The body burns fat for energy and loses extra fat. Losing excess fat translates into numerous health benefits. Insulin is a hormone required to drive glucose into the cells. Insulin levels are adjusted to meet the amount of glucose in the blood, i.e., higher after meals and less between meals since insulin is empty after every meal. Insulin levels are high most of the time throughout the day.

Due to insulin anesthesia, high insulin levels can be stabilized, causing insulin anesthesia— prediction and diabetes type 2. Fasting helps to keep insulin levels low, this reduces the risk of diabetes. Fasting also has a beneficial effect on the brain. It challenges the mind in the same way that physical or cognitive exercise does. It promotes the preparation of neurotrophic factors, which support the growth and survival of neurons.

However, fasting for all. Among those who try to fast are: - Children and adolescents - Pregnant or lactating women - People with eating disorders, diabetes type 1, advanced diabetes, or some other medical problem - overweight or the weak can be fasting unsafe, or if not done correctly.

There are various approaches to fasting intermittently. But the easiest thing to achieve is probably one that only enhances your daily routine. A regular 16-hour cycle followed by an 8-hour meal window is usually lasting. From time to time, fasting to be safe and effective fast, it should be combined with balanced foods that provide proper nutrition.

Staying hydrated, and knowing your physical limits while fasting is essential. The fast should break slowly. Avoid eating unhealthy foods, especially after fasting.

What Is Intermittent Fasting?

The concept of intermittent fasting suggests that you would skip one or more meals in a row to tap into your body fat stores to burn off your body fat and to achieve a higher level of metabolic flexibility. That is, you're going to use these periods of not eating to repair your body to upregulate enzyme systems that pull the fat out of storage to build more mitochondria, which is where the fat burns.

The idea of intermittent fasting was initially more extended periods a day. At least in my estimation, 24 hours is probably the minimum of what I would call intermittent fasting. Now a lot of people are using the term intermittent fasting to apply what I would call occasional eating, which is a compressed eating window, so for instance. I generally eat from 1:30 in the afternoon until 7 p.m. I don't eat consistently to about eat two meals a day instead of three, and those are the meal times that give me 18 to 19 hours a day.

Where I'm not eating and where my body is undergoing all of these tremendous metabolic changes. I get greater metabolic flexibility greater metabolic efficiency. I'm burning off my stored body fat. I'm entering a period of what we might call a tapa G where the cells start to some housekeeping and housecleaning, all of which are contemplated to address an arena where we might be looking at longevity or more significant health or reduction of risk for certain diseases of civilization.

So, the idea of fasting intermittently again it's sort of up to the person like. I like to go at least a day without eating before. I call that intermittent fasting; otherwise, I call it a compressed eating window. The beauty of having established metabolic flexibility is that you don't suffer from skipping a meal or two or three in a row the idea is that if you're that good at taking fat out of your stored - body fat and combusting it for energy your body doesn't care where the power came from doesn't care whether it came from a plate of food or where they came from your hips or thighs.

That one of the most empowering things about this concept of metabolic flexibility is that you can go long periods without eating and have zero negative impact on your energy on your mood on your muscle mass on whether or not you get sick. Even almost no effect on your hunger, so the long answer that I just gave is it's relatively easy to do if you've established metabolic flexibility if you've done the work if you've built the metabolic machinery to access stored body fat and to burn the ketones. I think intermittent fasting works for a lot of people, some people who have medical issues and would be well-served to do this under the supervision of a trained doctor. It would be people who you know who have diabetes or women who are trying to conceive.

You know people with diagnosed diseases of certain types. Indeed, they'd be well advised to work with a physician. But otherwise, for most people, it's worth a try to you know do a foray into intermittent fasting. I don't think there's a perfect fasting window. I think it varies from individual to individual. I know some people who have breakfast and then don't eat until the next breakfast a day. Later or till lunch a day and a half later. When I fast, it's typically, I go from dinner one night to dinner the next night, and a lot of times, it's not that I planned it. It's that it just happened like I had a long day. I got involved in meetings, or I was traveling. I only didn't find time to eat. I wasn't hungry. I didn't need to eat. So, I found myself going 24 hours without eating. Typically, I stick to a regular eating schedule, which is 1:30 in the afternoon for my first meal and 7:00 7:30 at night for my second meal.

I don't have any other than the two meals a day schedule that I sort of it here too. I'm very flexible in how I skip meals the easiest way to determine. You're ready to start intermittent fasting if you wake up in the morning, and you don't need to eat or if you can skip a meal without getting hangry. You find that you have enough energy to get you to know 7, 8, 9, and 10 hours through the day without eating or a whole night of sleep. Then waking up in the morning and not eating or maybe going to the gym and doing the workout fasted and not feeling hangry or feeling like you're going to pass out from work. You did those are all indicators that you're becoming better at burning fat. You're deriving the energy from your stored body fat, and you don't require a meal to top off your energy stores.

The Fasted State

During fasting, your hormonal stimulus is glucagon. Glucagon stimulates and regulates a lot of these pathways. What I'm going to focus on today is the flux of metabolites in the fasted state. I have drawn the primary tissues that are involved in the fasting response you have the muscle the adipose tissue liver and kidney during fasting you have 18 amino acids that go through transamination and primarily produce alanine, and glutamine alanine will go to the liver.

In the liver, alanine is converted to glucose. Glucose is then used by the rest of the tissues primarily by the brain. The brain loves glucose, and so it's a huge energy sink the other essential tablets that are used for gluconeogenesis will focus here on the adipose tissue. Adipose tissue during fasting triglycerides is cleaved to free fatty acids and glycerol. The glycerol is another substrate for gluconeogenesis and produces glucose during the fasting state. The fatty acids go to the liver, and the fatty acids are used to make ketone bodies.

This process is your fatty acid oxidation or beta-oxidation. The ketone bodies are a form of energy, and the liver releases them. The liver makes ketone bodies; it does not use ketone bodies if the brain and muscle mainly use ketone bodies. We've talked about the adipose tissue. We've talked about the muscle the one amino acid that I haven't finished with yet is glutamine.

Glutamine will go to the kidney, and in the kidney glutamine, the carbon backbones are used to make glucose through gluconeogenesis. But glutamine also releases ammonia. This ammonia is essential. I just told you that fatty acid is used to produce ketone bodies in the liver.

They're mild acids, so it's essential for the mild acids to be neutralized, and so the ammonia produced from tight glutamine rates. The acidity of those ketone bodies in the urine so glutamine does two things and makes glucose. It gives you vapor to titrate those ketone bodies, so in summary, then the big picture is other tissues contribute to the synthesis of glucose your muscle gives you amino acids and an amino acid alanine goes to glucose. The liver glutamine goes to glucose in the kidney the adipose tissue contributes glycerol, which is used for gluconeogenesis the free fatty acids are an essential fuel that'll go to the liver to make ketone bodies.

One important thing about the ketone bodies is that they're used in what's called fuel sparing if your body kept using those amino acids. Your muscles would be completely depleted, and the diaphragm is the most they're most susceptible to this. Therefore, the brain switches from using just glucose in prolonged fasting to using ketone bodies.

So basically, it switches from glucose to using fat because ketone bodies come from those fatty acids when it does this you need to make less glucose. Thus, gluconeogenesis decreases, and the proteolysis, the breakdown of your muscle decreases, and your body's protected as long as you have fat. You'll be excellent for a prolonged fast once you've depleted that fat. Unfortunately, you go back to using the amino acids.

Fasted and Your Metabolism

The human body has immense plasticity, the ability to adapt to unimaginable stressors to maintain homeostasis, a state of living that is no different when fasting abstaining from all nutritional energy that we receive from our macronutrients. How does it keep you alive when you do not consume food for days at a time? Does your metabolism change? How do your hormones change? I'll tell you we know that metabolism does not slow from something relatively mild like a 16-hour fast.

But after several days of no energy intake, your metabolism may decrease to compensate influenced chiefly by the decreases in leptin, which binds your hypothalamus, which controls your metabolic rate through actions like spontaneous movement. Which will reduce to pay for the lack of energy intake? As fasting continues, blood glucose sugar levels decrease before eventually leveling out. Decreases further substantiate this in glucose metabolism as the cells mostly begin to shift toward fat metabolism. Again, this is also evidenced as lipids fats are released from adipocytes fat cells to be taken up by other cells of the body and for the use in fat metabolism. Predictably ketones also increase as the liver begins converting lipids to ketones to fuel the brain and other ketone consuming cells.

Finally, many different amino acids change in concentration. But notably, leucine content skyrockets. Because of protein breakdown from degradation within the cells of the body. While I already mentioned leptin, the hormone glucagon increases, and insulin decreases as glucose decreases glucagon to stimulate gluconeogenesis, the formation of new glucose from the liver and kidneys releasing it into the bloodstream to maintain blood glucose. While insulin decreases as the pancreas does not get the stimulus to release insulin due to decrease blood glucose levels.

As a backup mechanism, cortisol also increases if the fast continues beyond several days. As cortisol further stimulates the release of a variety of substrates highest in the morning, finally, growth hormone also pulses throughout 24 hours increased at night to stimulate fat breakdown from the adipocytes. Overall you can fully expect a shift from a glucose centric metabolism to a fatter centric metabolism as a variety of hormones interplay to fulfill the overall result of keeping you alive and functional.

Fasted and Your Brain

Some of the ways the past thing can affect your brain and your mental health. I think you're going to love learning about what the brain and the nerve cells are doing for you while you fast. There are two types of intermittent fasting try fasting and water fasting with water fasting; you could drink water. But in a dry fast, staying from both food and water and it's called intermittent fasting. Because it's done at regular intervals, both types of passing have a profound effect on how your brain works and even increases the production of nerve cells, and the mind is a pretty fantastic place.

We're discovering using some pretty amazing things, one of them is that during fasting, it kicks into gear and increases the production of certain substances. One of these substances is a protein called brain-derived neurotrophic factor or BDNF. This protein helps to keep the nerve cells working and growing. But it also enhances their function. It improves brain circuitry increases the production of nerve cells that protects the brain cells from premature death. It also increases what is known as brain plasticity brain.

Plasticity is the brain's ability to create new pathways that give you many benefits, including adapting and learning needs E&M essentially helps to rewire your brain. This brain plasticity happens even at the level of the synapse.

What Is the Synapse?

A synapse is a junction between nerve cells that allows for impulses traveled from one nerve to the nest BDNF controls excitability and regulation at the synaptic level. We can modify our responses to certain stimuli. Our events started Belington, our mood, depending on the situation. We can control our feelings better by either reducing or increasing the chemical response at the level of the nerve cell to adapt to our environment.

It also helps with learning memory and focusing on a task, so what else does BDNF do it combat a process called excitotoxin city in the brain. You might have guessed excitotoxin city isn't a good thing, so what is it exciting toxicity is the process in which neurons are damaged and killed by over activation of nerve cell receptors in the brain. Under normal circumstances with healthy brain cells, chemicals known as neurotransmitters are released at the level of the synapse.

This allows impulses or information to be passed from one cell to the next exciting toxicity causes overstimulation of the neurons due to excessive release of certain chemicals, and it damages and kills your brain cells in the process. What happens when there's a reduction in the BDNF well there's a correlation between low levels of BDNF and certain diseases low levels of BDNF are associated with neurodegenerative diseases such as Parkinson's disease Alzheimer's disease multiple sclerosis and high intense illness and even depression decreased levels of BDNF also have an effect on learning, and BDNF decreases with age there are several ways to increase BDNF.

Fasted and Your Muscle Mass

I want to talk about the connection between fasting and building muscle. It's not just about the fat loss when it comes to putting on the right muscle, and it has some benefits. And I'll leave that with the study of the Western Journal of Medicine. According to this research, it was done after three days of fasting. Keep in mind that this extension is fasting, not just intermittent fasting, but whatever they found, there was a three. One hundred and fifty-five percent increase in hormones of human development is excellent. Still, a different study published in the Journal of Endocrinology Metabolism found that the human growth hormone has increased fivefold by just one hundred-day fast. Now I'm talking about this before it sounds a bit like a broken record.

I'm always referring to the human reproductive hormone when it comes to intermittent fasting. I want to do is Explain how the human growth hormone is like the effect when it comes down to building muscle, you see that the human growth hormone is just Not random, it is a 191 amino chain, which means that it acts like a protein in the body that moves around it and now stimulates the development of different things.

The soma in the pituitary gland is generated by the cells and what chondrocyte cells say they are divided into the cartilage. Now you will be surprised what you have to do with the cartilage of the muscle. When these cells divide, they become dynamic. Collagen Synthesis and Collagen Production Collagen give structure to our cells when it comes to muscle. Well, the muscles help in growth and formation, but collagen is also going to help us do many other things like tendon.

In the power of this and everything like that, you may have noticed by now that anyone who goes to human growth hormone therapy or any type of anti-aging treatment usually ends up with good skin, which is why it's just the reason is that they have increased collagen production and collagen is also helpful in helping your skin, but when human pro-tan's down to protein. It does something special when you see that it has low protein oxidation.

So, we have two different things:

- Protein synthesis.
- Protein oxidation.

Where you are eating more protein, they are oxidized and eventually toxic, and then we have protein synthesis, which reduces the rate of protein oxidation in the human growth hormone formulation, which means you consume more protein are used. Therefore, when you are fasting, the human growth hormone increases five times. NG can be mighty when it comes to muscle building. Now let's talk about son hydroxybutyrate. I have spoken about beta-hydroxybutyrate when it comes to ketosis, but I don't always mention it when it comes to fasting you see when you go into fasting your body uses this ketone body. It manufactures what is called beta-hydroxybutyrate.

Now, beta-hydroxybutyrate does many things inside the body. But in this particular case, I want to talk about research that looked at players who were already in a ketogenic or fast-growing state of son hydroxy biotite, and their muscles when they were working. How did they affect the surface, did they see the athletes that had to work with while fasting, but they measured their son's hydroxybutyrate levels?

But then they measured their muscle cells. Take a look at some of the things they learned that the presence of hydroxybutyrate on their muscles increased the survival rate of cells means that you didn't burn muscle tissue every time you exercised while you were working if you smoked a little flesh. So, if the son hydroxy biotite, which is the result of fasting, helps the muscles to survive, that is a good thing. Still, the other thing that happened with this son hydroxy biotite was that he found in mitochondria—increased ATP function. This means that physically eating your muscles yes by eating and not working out. Also, given the increase is such amazing right muscle. If you hear about the meditation, then you are a limiting factor in muscle building if you have never seen these Belgian blue cows before with cows that are wholly united with their brains.

They look weird so that they can make genetic changes. Deficiency of myostatin means that their muscle is capable of growing in a high amount. There is a high level of myostatin in humans. Myostatin prevents our muscles from eventually increasing and the way it works, which is known as the auto cream function. Muscle cells are never found to be primarily blocked or eventually enlarged so that more and more mutation becomes less muscular and more muscular. There is a very complicated relationship. There was a study that looked at it, and the International Journal of Sports and Health found that test subjects who exposed to only a small amount of testosterone are on a large scale.

The significant decrease in their levels of metastases in many muscles means that it can only be used in certain parts of the body. I was not systemic. A slight increase in testosterone equals less somatostatin, which means that your body can exert as much muscle as you were genetically capable of before testosterone. But now we have to create a link between fasting and testosterone so that you can see the endocrinology of the European Journal that I have given a lot of references to. Studies have shown that fasting increases what is known as luteinizing hormone.

The luteinizing hormone is secreted by the pituitary gland, which ultimately produces more testosterone and equals more testosterone to latex cells. This is the first step in the equation. So, fasting is high. Increase testosterone by one hundred and eighty percent, and if we have an increase in testosterone, then we have a decrease in myostatin. And we're able to feel a lot better in the process So that you have a combination of human growth hormone metastatic and, of course, a beta-hydroxybutyrate, which is safe, puts you at a triple risk when it comes to being able to build muscle to protect your muscles.

Chapter 2

What is Intermittent Fasting and Why Would You Do It?

What is intermittent fasting?

Intermittent fasting refers to maintaining zero or very low-calorie intake periodically for a specified period. Cyclical means not always fasting. It can be one day a week or one day a month, but not for several days. This is very different from the traditional method of digging the valley or losing weight. Intermittent fasting generally means not eating for 18-36 hours.

Zero-calorie or very low-calorie intake is also different from the traditional Pigu. Some people who eat grains can eat fruits and vegetables, but intermittent fasting does not eat anything except drinking water and supplementing vitamins and electrolytes.

Many people feel a little scared when they hear about fasting. In fact, in ancient times and famines, people often ate up and down, often in intermittent fasting. High blood pressure and diabetes at that time were rare and not entirely accidental. Also, we often inadvertently fast intermittently in our daily life, but we do not pay attention to. For example, after dinner at six, sleep on an empty stomach at night, and sometimes some people do not eat breakfast until noon the next day fasting for 18 hours. Furthermore, sometimes we are busy with work and can't afford to eat. This is also intermittent fasting.

How to Perform Intermittent Fasting?

Intermittent fasting every day, for example: only eat between noon and 6 pm; eat three meals early in the morning and then fast from 6 p.m. to 7 a.m., or eat only twice a day as needed. Intermittent fasting every week, for example: fasting every other day, or 5: 2 (five days to eat regularly, choose two days to fast).

Intermittent fasting every month, for example, five days a month.

What Are the Benefits of Intermittent Fasting in Weight Loss?
- Reduce the risk of cardiovascular system disease and diabetes.
- Promote the body to use fat as an energy source to achieve the effect of weight loss.
- Significantly increase growth hormone secretion and promote metabolism.

Why Is Intermittent Fasting So Popular?

Intermittent fasting (from now on referred to as IF) is very popular in Europe and the United States and has multiple benefits to the body, such as increasing muscle and fat, improving immunity, helping the body detox, and even prolonging life.

Fasting is very natural. In primitive society, we often had to be hungry for a long time to eat the next meal. When you are sick, your appetite will be reduced, and your body is telling you to use fasting to speed up recovery.

The most common and feasible fasting method is too fast for 16 hours (including sleep time) and eats 8 hours (usually two meals). During the 16 hours of fasting, you can only drink water, tea, or pure coffee. For example, you eat dinner at 6 p.m., go to bed at 10 a.m., get up at 6 a.m. without breakfast, you have to wait at least 10 a.m. before you can start to eat, and you can eat at will during the 8 hours from 10 a.m. to 6 p.m. (Of course recommend healthy food).

A survey by the International Food Information Council Foundation found that intermittent fasting was the most popular dieting method last year. Recently, Jack Dorsey, the president of Twitter, claimed that he only eats one meal a day, causing a lot of attention on social media. Many people criticize this approach as being too extreme, but it is undeniable that this is the current trend.

Impact on Health

The human evidence for "intermittent fasting" is still weak, but more and more studies have found improvements in different health indicators in addition to weight, especially blood lipids. Besides, those studies also mentioned that "intermittent fasting" may have more unique metabolic benefits than eating less frequently.

The most impressive and most controversial of these health benefits is longevity. Fasting can restart some regeneration processes in the human body, and prolonging life by limiting calories has been demonstrated in some animal models, but not all. But keep in mind that those animals spend most of their lives either on a low-calorie diet or intermittent fasting. It is not known whether "intermittent fasting" can delay human life. Even if it can, which variant is most effective, it will take weeks, months, or years to make a big difference.

Assessing the potential metabolic benefits of "intermittent fasting" is a long-term process. As mentioned in a 2015 systematic literature review, preliminary evidence is promising, but strong evidence remains few, so more human research is needed before fasting recommendations are a health intervention.

What Happens to Your Body When You Have Fast 16 Hours?

Fasting is a new tendency in modern society. Every religion has a fasting rule because we believe that fasting encourages us to be able to pray and be closer to God. We develop the ability to focus on God through fasting, and therefore we experience deep spiritual insight. But the modern concept of fasting shows us that, because of the mental benefits, fasting can be useful to achieve the goal of health.

What Is the Post?

Fasting is a must in every religion. For example, in Islam during the Ramadan month and in many religious communities, such as Buddhist monks and nuns, who follow the rules of Vinaya and do partial fasting. This is the process by which an individual eagerly limits the intake of food or drink. According to medicine, starvation means an empty stomach for a couple of hours or after the complete digestion of one meal.

However, fasting is a method without food, including religious rituals, detoxification, cleansing of the stomach, etc.

What Happens to Your Body: Day 1-2 Energy Lose?

At the cellular level, several things happen that cause hunger and fatigue in this first step. When you eat regularly, your body breaks down glucose to get the energy necessary for normal functioning. While you are fasting, your body needs to produce sugar to generate electricity, so a process called gluconeogenesis begins. During gluconeogenesis, your liver converts non-carbohydrate substances, such as lactate, amino acids, and fats, into glucose. As your body goes into Battery Saver mode, your basal metabolic rate, or BMR, becomes more efficient and uses less energy. This energy-saving process includes lowering your heart rate and blood pressure. At this point, you may feel exhausted. However, if you last a little longer, part of this lost energy will return.

What Happens to Your Body: Day 3-7 Fat Burning Regimen?

When you consume a typical carbohydrate-rich diet, your body breaks down sugar and turns starch into glucose. Glucose is the primary source of energy for our bodies. However, when you fast or begin to suffer from ketosis, glucose levels become limited, and your body must turn to fat stores to get the energy it needs. Your body breaks down fat into glycerin and fatty acids. The liver synthesizes ketones using glycerol. Glycerin is broken down by the liver to get extra glucose, and finally, these ketones are used by your brain as glucose becomes less available.

What Happens to Your Body: Day 8-15 Healing Mode?

In the third stage, your body begins to go into a "healing mode." This healing process begins when your digestive system rests from the everyday stressors and toxins that it carries daily. As a result, less free radical enters your body, and oxidative stress decreases. On the other hand, fasting causes stress, which provides additional benefits. This kind of mild stress is comparable to the stress caused by exercise, which ultimately makes you stronger, and your immune system more stable.

The Benefits of Fasting: What Happens to Your Body When We Fast?

1. Fasting Improves Brain Activity

Many might think that this is a little strange, but fasting indeed speeds up the brain. Studies have shown that in the event of starvation, the energy of the human brain increases because it changes the specific functions of the cells and, at the same time, increases the production of the protein, which is responsible for the activation of brain stem cells to activate new neurons. It also protects brain cells to go through the changes that occur in Parkinson's and Alzheimer's.

2. Improves Peace of Mind and Spiritualism

When we talk about human well-being, we cover not only physical health but also mental health, because a healthy body and a healthy mind are the two main assets of any person to control the overall function of life. Fasting for religious rituals makes us experience joy and mental satisfaction, as it helps us approach the Almighty. To achieve this, we deprive ourselves of the comfort that gives clarity to our thoughts. Therefore, fasting is necessary to purify our souls.

3. Helps Regulate Eating Habits

The modern lifestyle has changed all areas, especially our eating habits. Many are addicted to fast foods that are readily available everywhere, and for this reason, they face stomach and digestive problems. Fasting is an age-old practice that helps to start a healthy eating habit in everything. Five to six hours of fasting between meals or intermittent fasting reduces the consumption of junk food and indirectly supports the digestive system to work efficiently.

4. Helps Detoxify the Body

The term "detoxification" means a lot that relates to our well-being. This is perhaps one of the most amazing benefits of the post, which directly improves our system. During fasting, the lack of food for an extended period lays glycogen, which was stored by the liver in the form of glucose. Our body begins to decompose fat and release accumulated harmful chemicals from fats into the body and thus eliminate them with the help of the kidneys, lungs, lymph nodes, and skin.

5. Helps with Weight Loss

I am sure that with the help of fasting, anyone can lose weight naturally without spending hours on training. Intermittent fasting or random fasting for several hours a day eliminates fat cells from burning for energy. However, those who are overweight adhere to a strict dietary rule, ignoring tasty food for a long time, but this only deprives them of a lot. People can eat at regular intervals of 5-6 hours, and they will follow fasting for the remaining hours. A few low-calorie foods will prove more effective. Fasting is a new tendency in modern society. Every religion has a fasting rule because we believe that fasting encourages us to be able to pray and be closer to God. We develop the ability to focus on God through fasting, and therefore we experience deep spiritual insight. But the modern concept of fasting shows us that, because of the mental benefits, fasting can be useful to achieve the goal of health.

Can You Lose Weight Eating 2 Meals A Day?

We are often told that skipping one of the three meals of the day does not work. But it is quite possible to lose weight by taking only two meals a day without endangering your health. Sometimes we think we take three meals a day when this is not necessarily the case. A cup of tea, a glass of fruit juice, a simple yogurt, or even a quick toast is not considered a real meal.

To slim down with only two meals a day, you can skip breakfast or dinner but never lunch. This is intermittent fasting. It is not a diet, but a food habit that you give to your body. In the beginning, you can start with one day a week, then two, and so on so as not to rush your body. You have the choice between eating only morning and noon or only lunch and dinner.

Important

If you want to lose weight, eat three meals normally. It is best to eat less (fruit, vegetables, rice soup) or not to eat dinner, especially after 8 p.m., you can't eat anything, and don't eat it.

Or if you eat two meals a day, breakfast and lunch, replace fruit with dinner. Although this method works, you must take good results when you see results (if your body shape has reached your expected goals). The rest of the time is to pay attention to diet, cannot eat anything oily.

Then teach you the cruelest trick, do not eat meat, eat three meals a day full of seven (after 8 p.m., you cannot eat anything, do not eat). It won't take long for you to lose weight. However, this method is recommended for fat people. If you want to stay in shape, you don't have to use it so hard.

Eating two meals a day may seem crazy to you, even impossible or too difficult to follow. It is not only possible, but it is also how we ate before. This is no longer the case today, but the first men spent their day looking for food, eating a big meal in the evening, and they certainly had no obesity problems.

You may have heard the term intermittent fasting. It is a way of describing the diets which oscillate between periods of feeding and periods of starvation. Eating one meal a day is considered a strict time-limited form of eating since most of the day is spent fasting.

How Can Just Two Meal a Day Help You Be Healthy?

The idea behind eating just one meal a day is to eat less simply. Once the body adjusts to eating only once a day, it turns your stored fat into fuel, and ultimately you lose weight and become less hungry.

Ashley Smith, a nutrition therapy practitioner in Berkeley, explains, "You can become more effective mentally and physically." "It may take a few weeks to go from" sugar burner "to" fat burner, "but that will be done, especially when consuming a wide variety of high-quality fats, whole / nutritious vegetables, and good quality meat."

The secret is to eat a very nutritious meal and eat until you are full. You can choose the time of day, but it's easier to eat at the end of the day. Most people lose weight with this diet without having to watch their portion sizes or count calories.

Can I Lose Weight by Eating Two Meals a Day?

Some diets claim that eating up to six meals a day boosts your metabolism and keeps you from being hungry. The only problem is that regularly eating throughout the day encourages an obsession with food and overconsumption.

It also makes it easier to exceed your daily calorie limits. The truth is that eating six meals a day doesn't have a significant impact on your metabolism. You're just going to burn ten more calories. Some experts claim that not eating for a while slows metabolism. And that's true. But it would take three days of fasting to have a noticeable impact on your metabolism.

It seems that the more you eat, the more you want to eat. Everyone knows that. This leads to an obsession with food and overconsumption. The opposite effect also occurs. The less you eat, the less you want to eat.

When you are trying to lose or maintain your weight, it is easier to lose weight by eating less often. Ultimately, eating six meals a day makes you want to eat more and more often.

It is not for everyone. Not everyone will be satisfied with just one meal a day. Some people prefer to distribute their nutritional intake throughout the day. Eating 2 to 3 meals a day will always bring the same benefits.

Some nutritionists warn against restricting food to one meal a day and remind that it can promote an unhealthy relationship with food.

Some nutritionists claim that restricting meals once a day can encourage an obsession with food. While this may be true for some, many people who have adopted this lifestyle notice a significant decrease in hunger and a healthier relationship with food.

What Are the Side Effects of Intermittent Fasting?

Intermittent fasting is gaining popularity, and many people hope to lose weight in this way. Why can it help lose weight? What risks might you face? "Live well," ask nutritionists to analyze. However, to date, studies on intermittent fasting have been small and short-term. The sustainability and safety of intermittent fasting are currently limited to six months.

It should be reminded that although intermittent fasting can reduce weight in some people, it is not a panacea for improving health. If you overeat or eat unhealthy foods during non-fasting periods, you will not lose weight.

Another risk is inadequate intake of vitamins and minerals, which can affect normal cell function, growth, etc. If you choose to implement this diet therapy, it is recommended that you pay attention to food choices when you are not fasting. You should eat nutritious, high fiber, low fat and sugar, and balanced food.

1. Hunger

If you usually eat 5-6 times a day, the body will expect food at the times you typically use it to eat. According to Stephanie, the presence of the hormone glycerin is responsible for hunger.

Usually, hunger peaks at breakfast, lunch, and dinner and is partly regulated by food intake. When you first start the fasting diet, glycerin levels will continue to increase, so you feel hungry.

"During the initial 3-5 days, it will feel awful, but there will be times where you reach the dining window and no longer feel hungry," Stephanie said.

Specialist in nutrition and weight loss as well as a certified cardiologist, Dr. Luiza Petre, advises beginners on a fasting diet to fight hunger in the first 1-2 weeks by drinking plenty of water.

It aims to make the stomach feel full, make us stay awake, and get used to putting something in the mouth. Within 30 minutes of waking up, at least drink about 250 ml of water. When hungry, drink another 250 ml. What the fasting diet will teach you is that what you think hunger is thirst or boredom. Drinking black coffee and tea can also overcome desire.

Besides, sufficient sleep needs, stay busy, and avoid strenuous exercise in the first few weeks, because these activities will increase hunger. Eat enough the previous day and eat enough carbohydrates, healthy fats, and protein.

2. Headaches

Because the body is getting used to a new eating schedule, headaches are widespread. Edward Vasquez, a YouTuber who talks a lot about fasting through his Fledge Fitness account, provides tips for running it.

According to him, dehydration is one of the main factors. So, make sure you drink lots of water during fasting and meal times. According to Stephanie, headaches can also be caused by decreased blood sugar levels, and stress hormones released by the brain when fasting.

Over time, the body will get used to the new eating schedule. However, you try to be free from stress.

3. Lack of Energy

As a result of previously, you are accustomed to eating all day; your body may feel weak and underpowered because the body no longer gets constant fuel intake. Make sure you don't do many activities that consume too much energy, especially in the early weeks.

For example, avoid strenuous exercise and replace it with walking or yoga. Then, sleeping longer is also quite helpful.

4. Burning, Bloating and Constipation

The stomach will produce acids to help digest food. So, when we don't eat, we can feel like a burning sensation in the body. This can occur in the form of the discomfort of moderate-intensity throughout the day. This feeling will disappear over time.

So, keep consuming water, support our body to sleep, and avoid greasy and spicy foods because it can worsen the burning sensation. If the burning feels increasingly uncomfortable, consult a doctor.

Fasting diets can also cause constipation or constipation if the body is not hydrated enough so that it will cause bloating and discomfort. Stephanie suggests drinking plenty of water to overcome these problems and can prevent headaches and make the body more energized.

5. Feel Cold

The tips of the toes and hands that are cold when fasting are common but positive. When fasting, blood flow increases to fat reserves or adipose tissue. This can help move fat to the muscles, which means it can be burned as a fuel for power.

Stephanie said the condition of decreased blood sugar would also make us more sensitive and more comfortable to feel cold. Fight the cold feeling by drinking tea, taking warm baths, using layered clothing, and avoiding being outdoors when it's cold for a long time.

6. Overeating

People who are new to the fasting diet will tend to overeat. This could be because they thought that the calorie size did not affect or because they were starving, so they were very excited to meet food.

Planning food to be consumed can help you maintain ideal food portions. "When the fasting period is over, we must be careful with eating portions. You may indeed feel like eating everything, but choose healthy food options," Stephanie said.

Note these symptoms usually only occur during the week or a maximum of the initial three weeks. To avoid this, you can do it gradually so that the fasting diet will feel natural and healthy. So that appetite decreases mental acuity increases, then waist circumference decreases.

Fasting diets are also not intended for everyone—for example, diabetics, pregnant women, nursing mothers, or children. People who have chronic diseases also need to see a doctor first before starting a fasting diet.

People who have a history of risk of eating disorders also need to avoid fasting in various forms. There are times when the side effects of the fasting diet should not be ignored.

Chapter 3

Women's and Men's Guide to Intermittent Fasting

Discontinuous fasting may be an eating wherein you abandon food for a selected measure of your time a day. To help you explore your day, here's a manual for a way to plan your dinners during discontinuous fasting. What's more, recollect: Although this eating plan is organized around once you eat, what you eat is so far significant. During the timeframes, when you're eating, you will need to consider solid fats, clean protein, and sugars from whole food sources. While fasting is often overpowering, particularly on the off chance that you haven't done it previously, irregular fasting can be significantly simpler than numerous different types of eating plans.

When you start your irregular fasting venture, you'll find that you feel more full and may keep the dinners you are doing eat basically. There are a few varied ways you'll quickly, so I separated all of the various plans beneath into apprentice, moderate, and progressed alongside a commonplace supper plan for each day. The blend of supplements will offer you the vitality you've got to enhance the benefits of your fasting venture. Make some extent to think about a person's food bigotries, and utilize this as a guide for your specific wellbeing case, and alter from that time.

Keep in mind; discontinuous fasting doesn't mean calorie-controlled, so make sure to eat as per your own caloric needs. If you're a novice, start by just eating between the long stretches of 8 a.m. also, 6 p.m. is a fantastic method to plunge your toes into the fasting waters. This arrangement permits you to eat each feast additionally to some the thought of irregular fasting is entirely not something for the foremost part recommended for end of the day weight reduction. As indicated by Michael Wosley, restorative columnist and creator of The Fast Diet, he was initially suspicious of the technique, as well.

Nonetheless, following a time of research and playing guinea pig together with his eating routine, Wosley lost around 9 kg and a fourth of his muscle to fat ratio and has since been spruiking the benefits of fasting. A day of fasting may include something just like the accompanying: for breakfast, a dish (before the toast), berries and a tablespoon of yogurt, or ¼ cup heated beans on toast. Lunch could incorporate a touch plate of mixed greens with fish, egg or grains, and dinner could be something sort of a little pan-fried food, salmon and vegetables, or another serving of mixed greens.

It unquestionably sounds feasible; be that because it may, nibbling within the middle of dinners would presumably set you over as far as possible, so just in case you are a nibbler, it'd be increasingly troublesome. Wosley himself deals together with his fasting days by having a 300 Calorie breakfast at 7 a.m. (300 Calories being what could be compared to 2 cuts of light bread and a couple of boiled eggs), and afterward not eating again until his 300 Calorie dinner at 7 p.m.! Merely the thought of going 10 hours without eating makes my head turn, primarily as going this point allotment without fuel makes bound to cause a make a plunge glucose levels, bringing about that trademark shakes, even as an extreme diminishing focused and mental sharpness. Snacks yet at an equivalent time get in 14 hours of fasting inside a 24-hour term.

12 Health Benefits of Intermittent Fasting

1. May Bolster Sound Weight the Board

Via preparing your body to consume fat for vitality, discontinuous fasting can cash in of your body's regular weight reduction components. Additionally, the effortlessness of the arrangement implies you're substantially more susceptible to stick with it! At the purpose, once you practice discontinuous fasting and effectively switch your body into the fat-copying mode, your body is utilizing adrenaline to discharge put away glycogen and access fat to repeat. These expanded adrenaline levels can assist with boosting your digestion.

2. May Help Your Vitality

Not in the least like such vast numbers of calorie limitation eats less, which will cause you to feel lazy, the irregular fasting plan is meant to assist stable hormone levels with the goal that you're in every case effectively going to put away fat for vitality.

3. May Advance Mental Lucidity and Core Interest

Irregular fasting can help your intellectual competence since it expands your BDNF, which supports cerebrum network and new neuron development.

4. May Bolster Psychological Capacity

The hormonal changes that happen once you follow irregular fasting have been seemed to help memory and cerebrum work.

5. May Help Continue Solid Glucose Levels

Fasting can help bolster the support of typical glucose levels. While you're in your fasting window, no new glucose is being provided to your body, which means your organization must choose the choice to travel through put away glucose.

6. May Bolster Heart Wellbeing

Discontinuous fasting is an astounding supporter of heart wellbeing, in sight of its capacity to assist your liver's cholesterol creation at a substantial level.

7. May Bolster the Body's Calming Reaction

Your body depends on a procedure called "autophagy" to urge out old and harmed tissues and cells. At the purpose, once you quick and offer your body a reprieve from the consistent exertion of processing food, it's by all accounts able to concentrate more vitality on typical fix endeavors, which suggests supporting your body's natural mitigating reaction. Tons of research has been embraced on the impacts of fasting during the traditional Muslim month of Ramadan, wherein starvation happens among dawn and dusk.

One such investigation, which checked fifty people getting to initiate Ramadan fasting, included estimating the degrees of fiery master cytokines in their blood. Cytokines are particles coursing within the blood that react to changes within the host's wellbeing status. They could be genius incendiary, and enhance the side effects of constant sickness – as an example, interleukin 1 (IL-1), and tumor putrefaction factor (TNF) – or mitigating, and work to decrease irritation, and return the body to a solid-state.

During the fasting time of Ramadan, the members demonstrated diminished degrees of provocative expert cytokines within the blood, alongside diminished pulse, weight, and muscle versus fat ratio. These all expanded once typical eating was continued. Another fascinating finding was that immune cells were altogether brought down during fasting, anyway, because the proposed diet recommends just two days of irregular fasting. It's suspicious that insusceptibility would be smothered end of the day.

Another vital investigation looked to research the viability of irregular vitality limitation (same standards because the 5:2 eating regimen), with constant vitality limitation, during which lower calories were devoured a day. An aggregate of 107 moderately aged ladies was partitioned into the 2 test gatherings. Through the span of a half year, they were checked for changes in weight, alongside numerous different markers of wellbeing status. His investigation uncovered comparable outcomes for every gathering, with the two eating regimens prompting weight reduction, improved insulin affectability, and diminished cholesterol and circulatory strain.

These discoveries recommend that discontinuous fasting is often looked on as an appropriate option to full-time eating less food, unquestionably an alluring alternative for those not focused on going the whole hoard. One impediment to the investigation is that because it may, was that each member was urged to eat as indicated by a Mediterranean-style diet, which is synonymous with acceptable wellbeing with its accentuation on tons of plant foods and limited quantities of meat and dairy.

Food partition records, dinner plans, and plans were provided, which can well have driven members to receive an eating regimen ton more beneficial than their standard. Such an adjustment in eating examples may need improved their outcomes more so than the structure of diet they were embraced. Do you get suspicious once you hear people raving about another eating routine that creates weight reduction simple? We do not accuse you—body synthesis will generally be drunker than the consuming fewer calories industry leads on. In an industry loaded with contrivances and trends, there's one arrangement rapidly ascending to the bleeding edge since it's the heaviness of proof behind it.

An irregular fasting diet is progressively being lauded as an eating design that advances healthy weight the board while additionally being anything, but difficult to follow. Numerous people swear it is the most integral asset they've found for weight control, and they are not envisioning things. Irregular fasting's mystery lies within the way that it moves your body from consuming carbs and sugar for fuel to consuming fat. A recent report exhibited that this arrangement could help diminish your weight by 3-8% in 3-24 weeks! We've recognized a few key reasons concerning why discontinuous fasting for weight reduction works so well.

8. Clear-cut Advantage for Managing Cravings

Taking under consideration that the minor word "fasting" can cause us to feel hungry, it is lovely amazement for a few discontinuous fasting adherents to seek out that, after around 1-2 weeks, they nevermore experience many cravings for food during their fasting windows. Furthermore, no, it isn't only a stunt of the psyche or extraordinary resolution. There is a logical motivation behind why this happens. One of the foremost significant impacts that discontinuous fasting has on your body is that it underpins stable glucose levels. Normal glucose levels mean fewer sugar desires.

The other cool thing that happens once you start discontinuous fasting is that it underpins substantial degrees of a hormone called "ghrelin." Ghrelin is understood because of the yearning hormone. At the purpose when it's askew, that's the purpose at which you are feeling hungry constantly. Following two or three weeks of irregular fasting and stable ghrelin levels, you'll begin to ascertain decreased food cravings.

9. Common Calorie Restriction, But Better

At the bottom of just about every eating routine known to man is the idea of calorie limitation. We've all observed the recipe: Calories are eaten < calories consumed = weight reduction Calorie limitation is likewise the first motivation behind why most weight control plans flop over the end of the day. It conflicts with human instinct, and along these lines is fantastically hard to support. Irregular fasting has earned massive applause by the way that it usually prompts calorie limitation, without feeling like that's what you're doing. We wish to call it "slippery" calorie limitation. Here's the reason: a run of the mill discontinuous fasting plan (eating just among early afternoon and 8:00 p.m). typically compares to skipping breakfast. Since it's hard to dine in more than a selected number of calories per feast, cutting your day from 3 dinners right down to 2 can have a noticeable impact after a while.

Studies are finished watching a gathering of individuals who were approached to confine their calories throughout the day, and another collection that was approached to follow an irregular fasting plan. Both groups determined comparative medical advantages, except the discontinuous fasting bunch, experienced progressively bolstered glucose levels. In particular, the illegal fasting bunch discovered their eating regimen significantly more sensible. For the higher a part of us, it's mentally and naturally simpler to limit our eating to a selected period, rather than to confine our general day by day caloric admission.

10. Hold Lean Muscle Mass

Maybe the best drawback of the many confined calorie abstains from food is that they need to have been demonstrated to prompt loss of slender bulk, which hinders your digestion. This is often downright terrible news for your capacity to stay up any weight reduction.

The uplifting news? Research has indicated that irregular fasting causes you to hold fit bulk while so far shedding pounds. Phew!

11. Better Eating Habits

At the purpose, once you irregular quick, you will be adhering to a littler eating window than you presumably won't. This may typically eliminate late-evening eating, which is often a shrouded culprit of overabundance calories and subtle weight gain. At the purpose, once you realize that yielding to the munchies is just getting to show yourself out of fat-consuming mode, it is a lot simpler to oppose that late-night cooler attack!

12. It's Sustainable

Maybe the most striking aspect concerning the discontinuous fasting "fever" is that folks are treating it less sort of an eating routine and progressively like a way of life. Such vast numbers of adherents get themselves getting healthier, yet feeling much improved and wanting to stick with this eating plan. So discontinuous fasting can immediately become how of life change, rather than an accident diet.

Chapter 4

Styles of Intermittent Fasting

What Does "Healthy" Mean to You?

For me, being healthy methods having the option to do the things you love while you feel your best. So, wellbeing for you is characterized by having the opportunity to do the things you love. What do you like to do, and how does that work with your method for eating? I love being dynamic, regardless of whether that is through a turn or lifting loads or having the option to travel. I need the opportunity to do each one of those things without feeling like my wellbeing or my body keeps me away from taking a stab at something I might want to attempt. Presently, I've generally been moderately healthy; however, I believe that irregular fasting has helped me improve my decisions. At the point when I feast prep, I consider lunch and supper and perhaps a bite. I don't stress over breakfast or heft around a ton for a day of eating. In actuality, it's only one colossal holder.

What Eating Style Encourages You to Feel You're Most Advantageous?

I have joined a few eating styles. I began discontinuous fasting, Paleo, eating less gluten, eating more vegetables, and supper preparing in 2015. I found Whole30 in 2019, and I, at present, do a blend of the entirety of the above in my way of life. Whole30 and discontinuous fasting have most affected my healthy dietary patterns.

I regularly begin to eat around 11 a.m. or then again at noon, contingent upon my lunch plan at work. I have a generous lunch, and I'm commonly not ravenous until supper. I eat at around 7 p.m. I quit eating around 8 p.m. or, on the other hand, at 9 p.m. That is a 14-to 16-hour fasting window. In the early morning, I drink dark espresso and water, and that is it.

Generally, I'm still Paleo. Discontinuous fasting permits me to be somewhat more adaptable to what I eat and when I eat. I feel my best when I'm eating in a Paleo and Whole30 way (which, for me, implies, I limit my admission of handled nourishment).

What Were Your Objectives When You Rolled Out These Improvements?

I needed to have more vitality, improve my enthusiastic wellbeing, and feel less tired by and large. I needed to settle on eating and drinking decisions dependent on how this would fuel my body, brain, and soul as opposed to considering nourishment to be either positive or negative.

Did You Beforehand Consider Nourishment to be Nourishment Decisions as Either Positive or Negative?

Indeed, particularly toward the start of finding out about sugar, gluten, and dairy. I figured it was all bad, and all needed to be avoided. Presently I don't expand these fixings to such an extent, but not because that I consider them to be terrible; they don't cause me actually to feel so incredible. It's a slight move. It's generally about how I would feel right if I don't eat this or do eat that.

Everything being equal, I'll eat high-quality pasta and, I'm alright with feeling sluggish for the remainder of the day; however, I don't consider that to be as fortunate or unfortunate. It's precisely what's beneficial to me and how it will influence me generally speaking. Another model is I will have a go at everything when I travel. That is encouraging my passionate wellbeing and my social wellbeing and takes need over clean eating regularly.

16/8 Method

It is not a diet; it is a type of intermittent fasting or time-restricted eating. During this, you can't only eat low calories food, but you can also eat a variety of food in this you spend 16 hours of each day consuming nothing but unsweetened beverages like water, coffee, and tea. But remaining 8, you are allowed to eat anything by doing this. You can get many benefits like you can lose your belly fat and get smarter.

Do You Have to Do 16/8 Every Day?

We should try this method every day because it's beneficial for us.

Is It Helpful or Not?

Helpful fasting generally includes abandoning nourishment for a few days. On account of discontinuous fasting, then again, taking regular breaks from eating is adequate. However, is this methodology compelling regarding the members' weight and digestion? What's more, what does science need to state about it? For numerous individuals, another year commonly implies making goals.

Getting thinner is one of the most critical objectives, and there's no deficiency of chances to do as such, as counting calories methodologies flourish. Be that as it may, these frequently call for surrendering specific sorts of nourishment, a methodology that is unreasonable for some over the long haul. Interim fasting speaks to an alternate method for handling muscle versus fat. It's unique about slimming down in that it doesn't concentrate on changing what you eat, but instead basically deferring when you eat and are taking longer, regular breaks from eating.

Anna Engler found this pattern for herself and has just shed more than 30 pounds. She has been fasting utilizing the 16:8 techniques for a year now, which includes abandoning potent nourishment for 16 hours while drinking just dark espresso, tea, and water. Eating is permitted during the remaining eight hours of the day. "I don't need to skip pizza or Turkish fringes, which are my top picks," says the Berlin occupant. Engler enjoys a reprieve from eating beginning at dinnertime until lunch the next day. She says she discovers this mood to keep up, as she never especially enjoyed having breakfast in any case.

For a long time, Engler struggled with low motivation, a lack of discipline, and excessive weight. The 32 years old was significantly overweight but did not have any appetite for diets. "I always thought they were pointless because you gain back anything you have lost right away," she says. "This seems to be a method that is relatively easy to integrate into your day to day life without causing a lot of upheavals," Says Stephen Herzing. He heads up the institute for diabetes and cancer at the Zentrum vision, and he and his team conduct research into the ways that overnight fasting affects metabolism interval fasting have many other positive effects in addition to helping people lose weight. It also makes insulin more useful again,

For example, moreover, it lowers blood pressure and prevents cardiovascular disease over the long-term, and also supports cancer treatment. Together with his team, the researcher is currently exploring the questions of how fasting can be used for therapy purposes and how drugs that imitate fasting can be developed.

5/2 method

What is the 5/2 method?

It is a type of fasting in which we eat about 25% of our total calories that are required for our bodies. Usually, we needed almost 2000 2100 calories for two days, but in this, we only consume 500 to 600 calories. When we consume low calories, it helps to reduce our weight.

How Does It Work?

I am beginning the 5:2 Diet to shed a couple of pounds. We found out about it from my better half's sister, who shed more than 20 pounds in only a few months, so my significant other chose to check it out. I'm not a colossal fanatic of diets. I believe it's increasingly about "eating less and practicing more," yet that doesn't appear to be working, so I wouldn't fret taking a stab at something new.

Like a decent spouse, when my significant other beginnings an eating routine, I attempt it to check whether it can work for me. Makes feast arranging a lot simpler. So, as I'm expounding on this moderately new eating regimen, I'm somewhat eager since today is one of my two low-calorie consumption days.

Fundamentally, the 5:2 Diet lets you eat like you regularly accomplish for five days per week; however, then eat a low, low-calorie diet (nearly fasting) on the other two days. For my significant other, this implies only 500 calories for her and 600 calories for me. I'll get into the fundamental reasons in a minute; however, you can peruse Gina Crawford's book (and it will take you around 30 minutes).

Who Found It?

As indicated by Gina Crawford, Dr. Michael Mosley is the "organizer of the 5:2 Diet" and creator of The Fast Diet that I'm speculating broadly expounds than Ms. Crawford's guide for amateurs. Conceived in India, Dr. Mosley is currently a BBC TV columnist who produces appears on medicine and science.

After a short financial vocation, Mosley chose to turn into a specialist and learned at the Royal Free Hospital Medical School. Directly after he moved on from therapeutic school in 1985, he turned into an associate maker student for the BBC. It was in 2012 that he was credited with advancing the 5:2 Diet.

14/10 Method

14:10 requires you to fast for 14 hours and eat all your calories within 10 hours each day.

What happens when you don't eat for 14 hours?

During a 14-hour fast, you can expand without calorie refreshments. At the point when the 14-hour time frame is finished, you can continue your regular admission of nourishment until the following fast.

Notwithstanding weight misfortune, irregular fasting can positively affect your digestion, support cardiovascular wellbeing, and that's only the tip of the iceberg. It's protected to utilize this methodology on more than one occasion per week to accomplish your ideal outcomes.

Even though this procedure may appear to be simpler than curtailing day by day calories, you may get yourself very "hungry" on fasting days. It can likewise cause extreme symptoms or intricacies in individuals with particular wellbeing conditions.

You ought to consistently converse with your PCP before going on a fast. They can prompt you on your advantages and dangers. Continue pursuing to find out additional.

You'll be very much into your 14-hour time span before your body understands that you're fasting. During the first eight hours, your body will keep on processing your last admission of nourishment. Your body will utilize put away glucose as vitality and keep on working as if you'll be eating again soon.

After eight hours without eating, your body will start to utilize put away fats for vitality. Your body will keep on using put away fat to make vitality all through the rest of your 14-hour fast.

Fasts that last longer than 14 hours may lead to your body to begin changing over put away proteins into vitality.

24 Hour

Playing out a 24 hour fast can be a terrifying idea, yet with the correct tips and plan, you can effectively endure your fast. With this article, you will figure out how you can make it to 24 hours without breaking your fast, and find out about the advantages of fasting.

Since graduating from school, I've been hoping to try and investigate better approaches to carry on with my life without limit. Dietary patterns are one region I've concentrated on over the number of years, and specifically, trying different things with discontinuous fasting has led to some fascinating outcomes.

Regularly, I've adhered to an entirely loosened up 16-hour fasting window and 8-hour encouraging window since beginning discontinuous fasting, however now and then, I do a 24 hour fast (and once I did a 48 hour fast!)

On the off chance that you have never fasted, moving toward a 24 hour fast may appear to be a gigantic errand to take on. At the point when I began, I scarcely could make it past 9 a.m. before I "required" to eat. Presently, following a couple of long stretches of training, I once in a while, eat before 9 a.m.

Possibly you are interested in fasting and need to investigate your association with nourishment. It's conceivable you are hoping to get more fit and need to check whether fasting; merits giving a shot.

Whatever your explanation, I trust this post gives the data you need and need concerning fasting. Right now, I will discuss the advantages of starvation and share with your various tips for you to apply on the off chance that you are keen on a one day fast.

The Warrior Diet (The 20 Hour Fast)

The Warrior Diet is a method for eating that cycles broadened times of little nourishment admission with short windows of gorging. It has been advanced as a powerful method to get more fit and improve vitality levels and mental clearness. However, some wellbeing specialists contend that this fasting strategy is extraordinary and extravagant.

You can play out a 20-hour fast at whatever point you pick. You need to ensure that you get ready for your fasting day ahead of time. Eating healthy and balanced dinners before the fast will enable your body to traverse the 20-hour time frame.

A few nourishments you ought to consider eating preceding a fast include:

- Nourishments are wealthy in protein. For example, nut spreads and beans.
- Dairy items low in fat. For example, low-fat yogurt.
- Leafy foods.
- Entire grain starches.

Nourishments high in fiber will enable your body to feel full long in the wake of eating. Leafy foods contain water, giving you more hydration.

Drink water and other without calorie refreshments during the fast, yet remember that drinks with caffeine may make you lose more water. Drink an extra cup of water for each energized food to help balance your admission.

Keep on eating healthy after your fast is finished and abstain from indulging when it's an excellent opportunity to eat once more. You might need to have a little bite or eat a light supper when your fast finishes to assist you with moving to go into your standard eating schedule.

Alternate Day Fasting

It is a form of intermittent fasting, which involves fasting one day and eating the next and repeating this process.

A caloric limitation is a well-reported approach to get thinner, improve heart wellbeing, and conceivably even slow maturing. However, researchers, despite everything, don't concur on the ideal method to not eat.

New research in the diary Cell Metabolism plots a novel method to discontinuously confine calorie admission, a strategy that accomplishes similar medical advantages while potentially being more reasonable than continually limiting calories.

In a paper distributed on Tuesday, a worldwide group of scientists displayed the aftereffects of a clinical preliminary where "interchange day fasting" brought about diminished calorie admission, decreased weight record, and improved middle fat structure. Known as "ADF," it is a diet routine where followers maintain a strategic distance from all nourishment and caloric drinks for 36 hours, at that point eating whatever they need for 12 hours—doughnuts, treats, dumpster pizza, whatever.

Right now, preliminary, 30 non-corpulent volunteers who had done ADF for in any event a half year were contrasted over four weeks with 60 healthy control subjects. While the consequences of this clinical preliminary show that ADF had comparative medical advantages to caloric limitation, even though the "feast days" could incorporate a ton of unhealthy calories. The specialists additionally compose that ADF has some unmistakable preferences over CR. For the most part, they state it might be simpler to keep up the propensity.

"Here, we appear in a clinical preliminary that a related mediation, interchange day fasting (ADF), additionally leads to a striking decrease in by and large calorie admission throughout the investigation however is more effectively endured than consistent CR and incites comparable helpful changes on the cardiovascular framework and on body piece while being ok for a time of >6 months," compose the examination's creators, drove by first creator Slaven Stankovic, Ph.D., a postdoctoral scientist at the University of Graz in Austria.

"We likewise discovered positive modifications in cardiovascular illness chance variables and fat mass after just a month of ADF. Later on, this training, which is as of now developing being used as a way of life mediation, could, in the long run, oblige present-day social insurance in different settings."

Past work on discontinuous fasting has demonstrated that confining a creature's calories—without denying them satisfactory sustenance can expand their life expectancy. However, a significant part of the work has been constrained to monkeys and other non-human creatures.

This most recent examination expands on that current research by following a fair-sized human partner for sufficient opportunity to show critical advantages as well as no adverse symptoms.

The Two "RULES" Alternate Day Fasting

You can drink sans calorie refreshments on fasting days like unsweetened coffee and tea, water, and so forth.

You can eat up to 500 calories or 20-25% of your vitality prerequisites on fasting days.

Chapter 5

Transitioning into Intermittent Fasting (Switch Style)

Transitioning into the 16/8 Method

What Is 16/8 Intermittent Fasting?

It is not a diet; it is a type of intermittent fasting or time-restricted eating. During this, you can't only eat low calories food, but you can also eat a variety of food in this you spend 16 hours of each day consuming nothing but unsweetened beverages like water, coffee, and tea. But remaining 8, you are allowed to eat anything by doing this. You can get many benefits like you can lose your belly fat and get smarter. We should try this method every day because it's beneficial for us. Helpful fasting generally includes abandoning nourishment for a few days. On account of discontinuous fasting, then again, taking regular breaks from eating is adequate.

However, is this methodology compelling regarding the members' weight and digestion? What's more, what does science need to state about it? For numerous individuals, another year commonly implies making goals. Getting thinner is one of the most critical objectives, and there's no deficiency of chances to do as such, as counting calories methodologies flourish. Be that as it may, these frequently call for surrendering specific sorts of nourishment, a methodology that is unreasonable for some over the long haul. Interim fasting speaks to an alternate method for handling muscle versus fat. It's unique about slimming down in that it doesn't concentrate on changing what you eat, but instead basically deferring when you eat and are taking longer, regular breaks from eating.

Anna Engler found this pattern for herself and has just shed more than 30 pounds. She has been fasting utilizing the 16:8 techniques for a year now, which includes abandoning potent nourishment for 16 hours while drinking just dark espresso, tea, and water.

Eating is permitted during the remaining eight hours of the day. "I don't need to skip pizza or Turkish fringes, which are my top picks," says the Berlin occupant. Engler enjoys a reprieve from eating beginning at dinnertime until lunch the next day. She says she discovers this mood to keep up, as she never especially enjoyed having breakfast in any case. For a long time, Eager struggled with low motivation, a lack of discipline, and excessive weight. The 32 years old was significantly overweight, but did not have any appetite for diets. "I always thought they were pointless because you gain back anything you have lost right away," she says. "This seems to be a method that is relatively easy to integrate into your day to day life without causing a lot of upheavals," Says Stephen Herzing. He heads up the institute for diabetes and cancer at the Zentrum vision, and he and his team conduct research into the ways that overnight fasting affects metabolism interval fasting have many other positive effects additionally to helping people reduce.

It also makes insulin more useful again, For example. Moreover, it lowers blood pressure and prevents cardiovascular disease over the long-term, and also supports cancer treatment. Together with his team, the researcher is currently exploring the questions of how fasting can be used for therapy purposes and how drugs that imitate fasting can be developed. To begin, start by picking an eight-hour window and point of confinement your nourishment admission to that time length.

Numerous individuals want to eat among early afternoon and 8 p.m., as this implies, you'll need to quick medium-term and skip breakfast yet can at present have a balanced lunch and dinner, alongside a couple of snacks for the day. Numerous people will reveal to you that it's not about the planning of your food; however, the way that you limit your food admission to an 8-hour timeframe. Yet, an ongoing examination distributed in the diary Cell Metabolism proposes that early time-limited eating (doing your fasting around evening time rather than the morning) has a medical advantage in any event when no weight reduction happens.

The examination utilized men with prediabetes and put them into two gatherings:

Early time-confined eating (6-hr nourishing period, with dinner before 3 p.m). Control bunch with a 12-hour eating plan the examination ran for five weeks. The TRF improved insulin affectability, β cell responsiveness, circulatory strain, oxidative pressure, and craving in any event when the members didn't get in shape. Be that as it may, they confined food consumption from 8 a.m. to 2 p.m. So, the examination utilized a 6-hour window rather than an 8-hour window. Remember that this methodology didn't prompt fat misfortune in all members. Fat misfortune has more to do with calorie limitation (don't accept people who reveal to you in any case) than whether you quick or not. In any case, it shows that there are medical advantages to irregular fasting/time-confined eating autonomy from weight reduction.

So, the most significant inquiry you have to answer when you follow an eating regimen or procedure like discontinuous fasting is, "Would I be able to make this into a way of life? On the off chance that you can't keep up an irregular fasting plan, at that point, you'll get results at first. In any case, you'll probably slide over into your old propensities as the irregular fasting plan turns out to be too difficult to even think about maintaining. The science concerning intermittent fasting is a starter and dubious because of a nonattendance of concentrates on its long-haul effects.

There is fundamental proof that discontinuous fasting might be successful for weight reduction, may diminish insulin obstruction and fasting insulin, and may improve cardiovascular and metabolic wellbeing, even though the long-haul manageability of these impacts has not been studied. The AHA suggests irregular fasting as a possibility for weight reduction and calorie control as a feature of a "purposeful way to deal with eating that centers around the planning and recurrence of dinners and snacks as the premise of a more advantageous way of life and improved hazard factor management."

For overweight people, fasting might be incorporated into a more extensive dietary change, for example, "putting snacks deliberately before suppers that may be related with indulging," arranging dinners and snacks for the day to help oversee yearning and control feast parcels, and "advance steady medium-term quick periods."

The AHA noticed that eating some food on a quick day (rather than a total ready) delivered the best weight reduction and diminishes in insulin opposition when in any event, 4% weight reduction was accomplished by fat individuals. The American Diabetes Association "discovered constrained proof about the wellbeing and additionally impacts of irregular fasting on type 1 diabetes" and primer consequences of weight reduction for type 2 diabetes, this doesn't prescribe a particular dietary example for the administration of diabetes until more research is done, suggesting instead that "medicinal services suppliers should concentrate on the key factors that are basic among the examples."

New Zealand's Ministry of Health thinks about that discontinuous fasting can be advised by specialists to certain people, aside from diabetics, expressing that these "diets can be as successful as other vitality limited weight control plans, and a few people may discover them simpler to adhere to" yet there are conceivable symptoms during fasting days, for example, "hunger, low vitality levels, unsteadiness and poor mental working" and note that solid food must be picked on non-quick days.

Transitioning into 5/2

It is a type of fasting in which we eat about 25% of our total calories that are required for our bodies. Usually, we needed almost 2000 2100 calories for two days, but in this, we only consume 500 to 600 calories. When we consume low calories, it helps to reduce our weight. I am beginning the 5:2 Diet to shed a couple of pounds. We found out about it from my better half's sister, who shed more than 20 pounds in only a few months, so my significant other chose to check it out. I'm not a colossal fanatic of diets. I believe it's increasingly about "eating less and practicing more," yet that doesn't appear to be working, so I wouldn't fret taking a stab at something new.

Like a decent spouse, when my significant other beginnings an eating routine, I attempt it to check whether it can work for me. Makes feast arranging a lot simpler. So, as I'm expounding on this moderately new eating regimen, I'm somewhat eager since today is one of my two low-calorie consumption days. Fundamentally, the 5:2 Diet lets you eat like you regularly accomplish for five days per week; however, then eat a low, low-calorie diet (nearly fasting) on the other two days. For my significant other, this implies only 500 calories for her and 600 calories for me. I'll get into the fundamental reasons in a minute; however, you can peruse Gina Crawford's book (and it will just take you around 30 minutes).

As indicated by Gina Crawford, Dr. Michael Mosley is the "organizer of the 5:2 Diet" and creator of The Fast Diet that I'm speculating broadly expounds than Ms. Crawford's guide for amateurs. Conceived in India, Dr. Mosley is currently a BBC TV columnist who produces appears on medicine and science. After a short financial vocation, Mosley chose to turn into a specialist and learned at the Royal Free Hospital Medical School. Directly after he moved on from therapeutic school in 1985, he turned into an associate maker student for the BBC. It was in 2012 that he was credited with advancing the 5:2 Diet.

The 5:2 eating routine, or The Fast Diet, is somewhat unique about most conventional, irregular fasting plans. Rather than declining food during any set fasting window, you instead drastically limit your calories for a while. In particular, you eat regularly for five days of the week. On the other two days (your decision,) ladies limit their calories to 500 for the afternoon, and men remain beneath 600 calories for each day. Genius: You never need to confront extensive periods where you're not permitted to eat anything. This is an extraordinary arrangement to slide your way into the idea of fasting, without making a plunge as far as possible. On: Two low-calorie days implies you do need to be entirely exact about checking calories two times per week, which can be a torment. That means you have to look into the caloric substance of all that you're eating, measure out your bit sizes, and keep track of the duration of the day.

Who it's for: People who appreciate the way toward tallying and following calories? (We realize you're out there!) This is additionally an extraordinary arrangement for any individual who is dismayed by the possibility of confronting cravings for food while fasting since you never really need to abandon food on this arrangement.

Monday & Thursday Fasting Days

If you choose to quickly on a Monday and a Thursday multi-week, you now need to accept to what extent you'll swoon for. You'll need ideally quick for 16 hours one after another, which has been seen as the sweet spot in fasting—you get the full advantages of a more extended fast without the challenges of finishing a more drawn out quick (contrasted with a prompt that continues for 24 hours or more).

Be that as it may, doing so might be trying with the 5:2 Diet since you separate your caloric points of confinement among breakfast and a night feast. In any case, you may think that it's more straightforward on your fasting days to get every one of your calories in a single treatment. It's truly up to you. The key is to mess with the fasting strategy for your picking; however, recollect, stick to one specific technique for a quarter of a year before you attempt another.

Wednesday & Saturday Fasting Days

By picking Wednesday and Saturday fasting days, you will not feel sincerely denied food and, subsequently, have a superior possibility of staying with the program end of the day. The 5:2 Diet is planned for getting prevent the emotions of hardship, tension, and blame that accompany such a significant number of regular diets. Fasting, no matter the technique that you pick, is never a standard eating regimen; it is a deep-rooted social change, and therefore the more you are doing it, the simpler and additionally satisfying it'll become.

The 5:2 Diet endorses two days of adjusted fasting and five days liberated from calorie tallying. When choosing which days during the week to quick, comprehend that you may be adaptable. What worked for you every week ago might not, due to social commitment or different commitments, work for you in the week?

The key is to select two nonconsecutive days during which to quick. So, as an example, on the off chance that you fasted on Monday, don't quickly again until Wednesday or later within the week, supplying you within any event one entire day between fasting periods.

Breakfast Ideas

A day of fasting may include something just like the accompanying: for breakfast, a dish (previous the toast), berries and a tablespoon of yogurt, or ¼ cup heated beans on toast. Lunch could incorporate a touch plate of mixed greens with fish, egg or grains, and dinner could be something sort of a little pan-fried food, salmon and vegetables, or another serving of mixed greens. It sounds attainable; be that because it may, nibbling within the middle of dinners would presumably set you over as far as possible, so just in case you are a slow eater, it'd be progressively troublesome.

Wolsey himself deals together with his fasting days by having a 300 Calorie breakfast at 7 a.m. (300 Calories being what could be compared to 2 cuts of light bread and a couple of bubbled eggs,) and afterward not eating again until his 300 Calorie dinner at 7 p.m.! Merely the thought of going 10 hours without eating makes my head turn, for the first part as going this era of your time without fuel makes bound to cause a make a plunge glucose levels, bringing about that trademark shakes, even as an extreme lessening in fixation and mental keenness.

Lunch Ideas

Grass-bolstered liver burgers are one among my preferred decisions for lunch during the week, and that they are incredibly simple to organize to possess during the entire week. You'll eat this over a bed of lifeless verdant greens with a primary handcrafted dressing for dinner full of B nutrients for solid methylation and detox pathways.

Dinner Ideas

Salmon may be a significant wellspring of omega-3 solid fats, and dark green veggies like kale and broccoli are high in cancer prevention agents. Salmon is one of my final top choices for its taste and supplement thickness. However, you'll choose any wild-got seafood that supported your personal preference. Serve nearby some of your preferred vegetables broiled in copra oil, and you've got a brisk and straightforward superfood feast.

Transitioning into 14/10

During a 14-hour fast, you'll expend without calorie refreshments. At the purpose when the 14-hour time-frame is finished, you'll continue your regular admission of nourishment until the subsequent fast. Notwithstanding weight misfortune, irregular fasting can positively affect your digestion, support cardiovascular wellbeing, and that is only the tip of the iceberg. It's protected to utilize this system on quite one occasion per week to accomplish your ideal outcomes.

Despite the very fact that this procedure may appear to be simpler than curtailing day by day calories, you'll get yourself very "hungry" on fasting days. It can likewise cause extreme symptoms or intricacies in individuals with particular wellbeing conditions. You need to converse together with your PCP before happening quickly consistently. They will prompt you on your advantages and dangers. Continue pursuing to seek out additional. You will be considered into your 14-hour time span before your body understands that you're fasting.

During the first eight hours, your body will keep it up, processing your last admission of nourishment. Your body will utilize put away glucose as vitality and keep it up working as if you will be eating again soon. After eight hours without eating, your body will start to utilize put away fats for vitality. Your body will keep it up using put away fat to form life during the remainder of your 14-hour fast. Fasts that last longer than 14 hours may cause your body to start changing over put away proteins into energy.

Early Eating Schedule

I, for one, practice this arrangement during the weeks' worth of labor. I'm not a morning meal individual, so I appreciate a few of cups of natural tea to start my day. Despite the very fact that you merely are skipping breakfast, it's so far imperative to stay hydrated. Attempt to, in any case, drink enough water. You'll likewise have natural tea, (Most specialists concur espresso and tea don't break your quick). The catechism in tea are seemed to improve the benefits of fasting by assisting with advancing lessening the craving hormone ghrelin, so you'll cause it until lunch and to not feel denied. Since you've expanded your fasting period a further four hours, you've got to make sure your first feast (around early afternoon) has enough healthy fats. The burger within the 8-to-6-window plan will function admirably, and you'll include more fats in together with your dressing or top with avocado!

Mid-day eating schedule

Nuts and seeds make incredible tidbits that are high-fat and may be eaten around 11 a.m. Splashing these heretofore can help kill normally happening proteins like phytates, which will increase stomach related issues. Have dinner around 2:30 p.m., and quickly like within the 8-to-6-window plan, a dinner with a wild-got fish or another clean protein source with vegetables is a fantastic choice.

Evening Eating Schedule

Fat bombs will control your appetite and provides you adequate sound fats to continue you until dinner. These are particularly fulfilling in light of the very fact that they need an aftertaste like cinnamon rolls.

Transitioning into 24 Hours Fast

Playing out a 24 hour fast is often a terrifying idea, yet with the right tips and plan, you'll effectively endure your fast. With this text, you'll find out how you'll make it to 24 hours without breaking your fast, and determine the benefits of fasting. Since graduating from school, I have been hoping to undertake and investigate better approaches to hold on with my life without limit. Dietary patterns are one region I've targeting over the number of years, and specifically, trying various things with discontinuous fasting has led to some fascinating outcomes.

Regularly, I've adhered to a wholly loosened up 16-hour fasting window and eight hours encouraging window since beginning discontinuous fasting, however now then, I do a 24 hour fast (and once I did a 48 hour fast!) On the off chance that you haven't fasted, moving toward a 24 hour fast may appear to be a significant errand to require on. At the purpose, once I began, I scarcely could make it past 9 a.m. before I "required" to eat. Presently, following a few long stretches of coaching, I once during a while eating before 9 a.m. Possibly you're interested in fasting and wish to research your association with nourishment. It's conceivable you're hoping to urge healthier and want to see whether fasting merits giving an attempt.

Whatever your explanation, I trust this post provides the info you would like and want concerning fasting. Right now, I will be able to discuss the benefits of fasting and share with your various tips for you to use on the off chance that you are keen on a one day fast.

Additionally, called an eat-stop-eat diet, a 24-hour quick included eating no food for 24-hours one after another, typically a couple of times for each week. So you'd get fast from dinner at some point until dinner the subsequent day. Or on the opposite hand breakfast to breakfast or lunch to lunch, contingent upon what you wish. On the off chance that you erode 7 p.m. tonight and do not eat again until 7 p.m. the subsequent day, you've quite recently finished a 24-hour quick.

Professional: This one is often exceptionally like a bustling day at work. Suppose you've got a furious day at the workplace or perhaps a whole day of movement. Instead of worrying about when and what to eat amidst your confused day, enjoy a reprieve. Try not to stress overeating throughout the day, until at whatever point, you come back home for dinner.

Con: you'd prefer not to do that one consistently. It isn't prescribed to try to a 24-hour quick quite twice hebdomadally.

Who it's for: People whose bustling timetables could profit by removing the pressure of discovering, preparing, gobbling, and tidying up food for an entire day, two or three days every week. With this type of IF, you quick at some point, eat the subsequent and rehash typically. There are two or three distinct approaches to try to it – a couple of strategies permits you to eat the maximum amount as 2000 kilojoules each day on quick days, while another interchange day fasting feeds less require fast days to be no-food zones.

The weight reduction results: consistent with a recent report that contrasted exchange day fasting with standard kilojoule-limitation consumes fewer calories; the eating regimens delivered an equivalent fundamentally as weight reduction results.

Stars: Like 5:2, supporters of interchange day fasting state the break between fasting days can make this eating regimen simpler to stick to than people who require day by day kilojoule limitation.

CONS: consistent with the 2017 investigation, the inverse may be valid – more people dropped out of the opposite day fasting diet than the day kilojoule-limited one since they were disappointed with it

Since consistently day should be a fast day, paying little mind to a way of life or social duties, this sort of fasting might not be as livable as others, which can clarify the above dropout rate.

Besides, an identical report additionally found that a half year after halting the eating regimen, interchange day fasters had raised degrees of cholesterol.

What to Eat to Interrupt Your Fast?

Breaking the fast in discontinuous fasting are some things that have got to be addressed. Irregular fasting is an eating routine arrangement which incorporates fasting and eating stage in regular periods. It's viewed as compelling in accomplishing weight reduction and furnishing your body with the essential detox. Fasting stage in irregular fasting can last anyplace between 10 to 12, 14, or 16 hours, contingent upon how you are feeling. An honest fasting window keeps going anyplace between 14 to 18 hours. Way of life mentor Luke Coutinho believes that you simply ought not to drive yourself to quick longer than your body permits. Start with 10 or 12 hours at the outset and afterward expanding fasting period by an hour during a week or three days.

During the eating stage, guarantee that you devour a balanced eating routine, so you get appropriate sustenance. Likewise, it's critical to affecting bioactive food is alluded to small biomolecules that are available in foods. They need the power to balance a minimum of one metabolic procedure, which thus are often helpful for better wellbeing.

Luke's plate of incorporate bioactive papaya, pineapple, watermelon, pecans and almonds. He says that these are crude bioactive, which may give the accompanying advantages.

- Angiogenesis - a procedure which inspires arrangement of fresh recruits' vessels.
- Undifferentiated cell insurance.
- Microbiome assurance.
- DNA assurance.

As indicated by Luke, everything of the above capacities can together assist in getting a stable insusceptible system. How you break the fast in discontinuous fasting for weight reduction.

Transitioning into the Warrior Diet (The 20 Hours Fast)

The Warrior Diet may be a method for eating that cycles broadened times of little nourishment admission with short windows of gorging. It's been advanced as a reliable method to urge healthier and improve vitality levels and mental clearness. However, some wellbeing specialists contend that this fasting strategy is extraordinary and extravagant. You can play out a 20-hour fast at whatever point you choose. You merely got to make sure that you prepare for your fasting day before time. Eating healthy and balanced dinners before the fast will enable your body to traverse the 20-hour time-frame. This includes fasting for a selected measure of your time every day, at that time eating whatever you wish during the opposite 'window.'

One of the foremost documented methods for doing this is often the 16:8 eating regimen: fasting for 16 persistent hours, at that time being allowed to eat during the opposite eight, with 10 a.m.-6 p.m. the foremost generally recommended 'eating window.' The weight reduction results: An investigation distributed in 2018 found that folks following the 16:8 eating regimen lost three percent of their weight in just 12 weeks since they ate 1400 fewer kilojoules each day, on faith them. Stars: thus far, check out proposes that time-confined eating plans, for instance, 16:8 could be more straightforward to remain with than different sorts of IF, maybe in light of the very fact that you can abstain from arising to be excessively eager.

CONS: Not having the choice to eat after 6 p.m. each and each day may confine your social and family life. And keeping in mind that you could also be enticed only to postpone you're eating window once you need to, specialists caution against it for best outcomes. I would conclude that I used to be getting to awaken at 5:30 ordinarily to exercise for a fantastic remainder. It's practically smart how frequently I even have done this type of thing to tumble off the wagon following seven days. These kinds of choices and this flawlessness outlook is 100% established in dread.

On the off chance that I can control my conduct, at that time, I can control my conditions and my life. Grasping firmly to control?? Look for the dread and manage it. At the purpose, once you can remove the fear in your life, you're opened to choose positive choices toward an objective, rather than attempting to accomplish the "objective" in one stage. On the off chance that model? Instead of going directly from a high-sugar, throughout the day eating way of life to a 20 hour quick, perhaps venture out moving breakfast back a few hours, or dinner up a few hours.

Early Eating Schedule

Papaya and Watermelon. Papaya is the ideal natural product for weight reduction. It contains stomach related chemicals referred to as papain, which may help in facilitating pharyngitis, improving absorption, mending wounds, and decreasing muscle irritation. It's useful for people with diabetes and may likewise help in promoting menstrual pain. Watermelon comes within the classification of hydrating foods, which will forestall the lack of hydration. It's low in calories and is impeccable to be remembered for a weight reduction diet. The natural product, which is in season during summer, is plentiful in vitamin A, vitamin B6, and vitamin C. it's likewise pressed with lycopene and amino acids - which may assist you with having unbroken skin and solid invulnerability.

Mid-day eating schedule

- ½ pound ground grass-sustained meat liver.
- ½ pound ground grass-sustained meat.
- ½ teaspoon garlic powder.
- ½ teaspoon cumin powder.
- Ocean salt and pepper to taste.
- Wanted vegetable oil.

Remember that this arrangement isn't for novices, and you need to consistently converse together with your medical care physician before beginning any fasting routine, particularly on the off chance that you merely are shooting up or have an ailment. It's prescribed that espresso consumers continue their morning espresso consumption, which everybody who does propel quickly remains appropriately hydrated.

Evening Eating Schedule

Eat good fats, clean meat sources, vegetables, and a few fruits. Even however, this arrangement is propelled, it's exceptionally straightforward. Try not to eat anything one another day. Each and each other day, eat good fats, clean meat sources, vegetables, and a few organic products, and afterward, on your fasting days, you'll expend water, homegrown tea, and reasonable measures of dark espresso or tea. With this data accessible, you ought to know precisely the way to plan suppers when beginning an irregular fasting plan.

Keeping in mind that it's going to appear to be confused from the outset, once you start fasting, it'll desire natural and fit pretty flawlessly into your days. Be that because it may, consistently start slow and steadily workout to further developed plans. It's likewise imperative to remember that you may have some "off" days when irregular fasting doesn't work for you. Tune to your body—on the off chance that you need to eat outside of your run of the mill window, it's OK! Restart when you are feeling much improved.

Chapter 6

Benefits, Risks and the Optimal Way of Breaking Fast

Intermittent Fasting and Its Benefits

The benefits to the brain, weight loss, and fitness make periodic fasting, an attractive option for anyone who wants to improve their health, especially for people with type 2 diabetes or those who are trying to maintain weight loss after obesity.

Slowed Aging and Improved longevity

The calorie restriction has received high pressure in the past few years for its role in increasing life expectancy in animal studies. Still, it is almost impossible to study the long-term restriction of food in humans ethically. Intermittent fasting triggers the same calorie restriction effects, so you get improved aging and a longer and healthier lifespan.

Promotes Brain Growth, Recovery, and Function

Intermittent fasting has several benefits for the brain. Tight regulation of your diet seems to improve memory, generate new neurons, improve brain recovery after an injury, raise your spirits, and reduce the risk of cognitive decline associated with aging.

Intermittent Fasting Regulates Hormone Levels

The levels of insulin, ghrelin, and leptin and the body's response improve with intermittent fasting. This means that your body is better able to respond to higher and lower blood sugar levels, as well as regulate hunger and satiety. Human growth hormone, a hormone that causes growth in children and helps regulate sugar and fat metabolism, also increases during cyclic starvation.

Intermittent Fasting Improves Blood Composition

Your body can better regulate the ebbs and flows of energy resources when you take a regular diet. Fasting, both lowering and somewhat ambiguous, helps maintain healthy blood sugar, blood pressure, insulin, and cholesterol. Improved blood composition reduces oxidative stress in the body.

Intermittent Fasting Reduces Oxidative Stress

Nutrition, as a rule, leads to oxidative stress, depletes your antioxidant defense against free radicals in your tissues. Intermittent fasting by its nature dramatically reduces your exposure to the inflammatory effects of converting food into energy because you eat less.

Intermittent Fasting Increases Fat Burning

Low insulin levels occur during fasting because you do not absorb a stable supply of glucose from the digestive tract. Low insulin levels stimulate fat-burning to maintain a steady energy level. Intermittent fasting gives you better access to your fat stores.

Intermittent Fasting Mimics the Beneficial Effects of Exercise

Sport training has many beneficial effects on the brain, heart, vascular system, stress response, and body composition. Intermittent fasting mimics many of the same benefits, such as reduced resting heart rate, improved immune function, increased DNA recovery, improved motor function, ketone production, increased stress resistance, faster recovery from stress, and enhanced disposal of old or malfunctioning cells.

Post Charts

As a rule, the longer the fasting period, the better the results. Some people find that they experience some emotional effects of fasting. You may find that you feel irritable and hot-tempered while adjusting to the intermittent fasting schedule.

Intermittent Fasting: Getting Started

If you can stretch your periodic fasting for more extended periods, you will quickly see lower levels of insulin and spend more time in ketosis, a fat-burning state.

To start intermittent fasting, we recommend starting with the 12:12 schedule: a 12-hour window where you can eat, and then a 12-hour fast. If you find this schedule simple, try program 8:16 onwards. Intermittent fasting for more extended periods with a relatively short meal period (6:18 or 4:20) is a critical component of the warrior's diet, a diet based on the eating habits of our ancestors.

Extend your post beyond this standard, and you will reach an alternative position. You must evaluate what works with your daily schedule and training goals to find a stable, steady, intermittent fasting regimen. Some fasting people think the fasting plan at 10:14 or 6:18 is better for them. In general, fasting will bring a lot of health benefits, so do not be afraid to change the schedule according to your needs. Just try to eat earlier in the afternoon and not late to reduce the accumulation of fat.

However, if you usually skip breakfast, feel free to start your meal around lunchtime. The physical impact of fasting on a person depends on innumerable variables. Some people respond to intermittent fasting significantly better than others. If you are experiencing unusual stress or experiencing some stressful life events, we would advise you to suspend your post until you cope with your weight due to the hormonal imbalance that usually accompanies (and nourishes) the reaction to stress.

Periodic Fasting - What Is During A Break?

Although you do not need to take another diet to try intermittent fasting, it is never too late to eat healthy foods. We recommend whole grains, a plant-based diet with lots of raw vegetables, fruits, nuts, and seeds to improve nutrition and maintain good health. If you want your food to contribute to fat loss, try ketogenic fasting.

Unlike most ketogenic diets or fasts, which are based on a significant amount of animal fat and protein to turn your body into ketosis, we have developed a plan to cleanse the body with whole plant foods. Such as avocados and walnuts, which contribute to healthy blood composition and reduce oxidative stress. In addition to burning fat reserves.

Does the 16/8 Diet Work?

The 16:8 diet is a type of time-restricted fasting done to achieve better health or lose weight. You will learn what the 16/8 food is and what rules you need to adhere to, losing weight in this way. The article will talk about the advantages and disadvantages of a diet, as well as how to improve the result. You will find out what you can eat on this diet and find out for how long and how many kilograms you can lose weight.

The number of diets and a variety of limiting nutritional systems is immense. Choose for every taste and color! Some are very tough and strict, such as the Japanese diet or the Maggi diet. Others are powerful and effective, such as protein or low-carb diets.

Some options are known throughout the world and by which even stars have been losing weight for many years - the Dukan diet. One way or another, there is no practical way to lose weight. No food would help everyone lose weight. Or is there any way?

Many people can involuntarily eat on the principles that will be described below. Diet 16/8 or interval diet is a way by which you do not limit yourself in any way and eat what you want, and at the same time, lose weight.

And in fact, the system is quite simple - this is the most common fasting! But the advantage is that you do not have to starve. So how does this diet work? Below you will find all the information about the principles of this method for losing weight.

Diet Rules

One way or another, before judging whether the diet will work or not, you need to understand its rules and find out why it is still so popular. The hunger strikes have long since become something completely ordinary for many people.

However, most of them do not approach this process correctly and can significantly harm their health. That is why the 16/8 diet is considered the most standard and relatively simple in the framework of the current reality. And the rules of the food are quite simple:

- Firstly, to sit on a similar diet, you must have an established schedule and sleep mode. Without this, there may not be results. Therefore, before you test your strengths through this method, think about how well you have a daily schedule. Think about what time you are most active, and what hours you rest and sleep. Based on this information, proceed to the next step.

- Next comes the most important - you choose the time for a hunger strike and the time for food. As mentioned above, you need to pick it based on your schedule. Think about what time you eat most often? Try creating a new plan so that your favorite mealtime does not disappear (even if it's the evening). But, of course, you can't eat anyway before going to bed a maximum of 2 hours before bedtime.

- An approximate graph may look as follows. You wake up at 8 o'clock, but you don't have breakfast right away. Let the body wake up, drink a glass of water on an empty stomach, take vitamins, and can-do exercises. After 2-3 hours, there will be the first meal.

- The report starts at breakfast. For example, you ate at 10 a.m., and now before 6 p.m., you will need to gain your calorie volume per day.

- After 6 pm, your fasting begins. Before going to bed, you can drink kefir or milk if you have time to get hungry, but it's better not to. With such a schedule, it is advisable to go to bed no later than 10-11 hours in the evening. Thus, you will not be hungry and will adhere to a regular sleep and diet.

Benefits

Many diets sound convincing and compelling, so most girls are always looking forward to this day with joy and embark on the active process of losing weight. But their hopes and dreams are shattered about cruel reality, because diets, especially strict ones, are crazy restrictions that neither the body nor the mind can be prepared for.

Each diet has its advantages and disadvantages. Below you will find several advantages that show this diet on the right side and can make girls think that it is beneficial and productive.

The Benefits of Diet 16/8 Are as Follows:

- Improved metabolism.
- Deep sleep.
- Stabilization of Eating Habits.
- Conscious consumption of food.
- Partially healthy nutrition.
- Lack of strict restrictions.
- Quick result.
- A simpler version for beginners (12/12, 14/10).

Disadvantages

But there are enough cons and problems with diets.

The Diet 16/8 Should Highlight the Following Disadvantages:

- Not everyone can withstand such a restrictive way to lose weight.
- Frequent hunger (first time).
- Rare but possible side effects.

- Prostration.
- Lack of mood.
- The risk of breaking and eating a lot of food in the allowed interval.
- The complexity of implementation for some people (for office workers, for example).

How to Improve Results

Of course, losing weight is a very long and complicated process, which must be approached comprehensively and wisely. Many people forget about the importance of proper nutrition on such diets, and when they see that there are "no restrictions," they allow themselves to eat fast food and drink all the food. And many other things are forgotten.

- Go in for sports (moderately) and do exercises.
- To drink a lot of water.
- Do not forget that meals should be filled with proper and high-quality food.
- Do not forget about eating vegetables and fruits.
- Try to maintain good spirits and believe that you will succeed.

Dates of Diet and What Results Can Be Achieved

Above, you could already see the information that there are different options for interval fasting. Indeed, there are harder ones, for example, 18/6 hours, and more relaxed, according to which, by the way, many live without even realizing it (12 / 12, 14 / 10).

If we talk about how much you can sit on such a diet, then everyone for himself decides whether this diet will be a test period, or whether he wants to make this diet a way of his life. One way or another, you need to stop the food only if you feel bad.

How Many Calories Should You Eat On 16/8 Diet?

The rules are simple - there are any products without restrictions, but only at certain times of the day. This diet, according to American scientists, can reduce not only weight but also blood pressure. And what do our experts say?

This diet is easy to follow. Experts say this study is the first to show the benefits of full access to food at one o'clock in the day and restriction of food intake at other hours in obese people.

Researchers at the University of Illinois at Chicago studied the effects of time-limited food intake in 23 obese volunteers whose average age was 45 years old, body mass index 35 (the formula calculates body mass index (BMI) - divide centimeters by body weight in kg per squared - $BMI = m / h2$, the norm is up to from 18.5 to 25.5 units). The results are published in the journal Nutrition and Healthy Aging.

Participants in the study could take any food in unlimited quantities between 10.00 in the morning and 18.00. However, during the remaining 16 hours, participants could only drink water or drinks that were almost free of calories. The test lasted for 12 weeks.

Compared with the control group, participants who followed the indicated diet consumed fewer calories per day, resulting in reduced weight and blood pressure.

According to the US Centers for Disease Control and Prevention, over the past few years, more than one-third of American adults are obese. It is known that obesity significantly increases the risk of cardiovascular disease and coronary heart disease and average working age.

The average teaching art studies nick 300 kilocalories consumed less, it possible to reduce the weight to 3%, and the blood pressure at 7 mm Hg, other indicators, including body fat mass, insulin resistance, and cholesterol levels, were comparable to those in the control group.

"The main conclusion of this study is that weight loss can be made without constantly counting calories or excluding certain foods from the diet," says Christa Varadi, author of the study, professor of kinesiology and nutrition.

Even though this is the first study on the 16/8 diet (16 hours of fasting and 8 hours of nutrition), Dr. Varadi notes the similarity of his results with earlier data on interval types of foods.

"The results we obtained were also observed in other studies that needed to fast for one day," says Dr. Varadi, "The obvious advantage of diet 16/8 is the ease of compliance. In our study, we observed fewer dropouts due to malnutrition compared with other trials."

"The preliminary data obtained in the study inspire confidence, but more extensive, long-term randomized trials are required," Dr. Varadi and colleagues say. "It is necessary to approach the selection of a diet individually since even a small efficiency of the method can positively affect the patient's health."

The opinion of The Diabetologist

The effectiveness of the 16/8 diet is related to when you go to bed.

"Such a diet will be effective only if several rules are observed," says dietician Elena Solomatina. - If you go to bed late in the evening, the body will have time to get hungry and develop high levels of insulin in response to low blood glucose. And waking up in the morning, you will want to eat something sweet, flour, and high-calorie, which, due to the high level of insulin, will immediately be deposited in the tissues in the form of fat.

If you go to bed earlier, for example, at 10 p.m., you will not have time to get hungry, and in the morning, you will not be pulled for flour and sweets. In this case, this power mode will work.

But this does not mean absolute "wild freemen" in food. To lose weight and maintain weight at a reasonable level, it is still essential to eat the same number of calories every day, eat a balanced diet, and go to bed on time.

How Can Reduce your Stomach Fat?

A flat stomach is the ultimate dream of many women and men. The problem of fatty deposits on the abdomen is prevalent. Even with a healthy weight, you can have a tummy. It is not so simple to remove the notorious stomach, but by following our recommendations regularly, you can achieve a significant effect.

Diet to Reduce Stomach

As much as we would like, we can't do without a diet. Fat deposits in the abdomen accumulate slowly, but correctly and mainly due to an unbalanced diet. Do not be afraid of the word diet. It is not necessary to limit oneself sharply in food and refuse favorite foods; you need to revise the principles of nutrition. Fiber-rich foods contribute to volume reduction.

It absorbs excess fats and excreted from the body along with other unnecessary substances. A lot of fiber is found in fruits, vegetables, legumes, and grains. You can use thread in the form of dietary supplements. In no case, do not refuse meat. But it should not be fat, but lean (chicken, turkey, rabbit, veal).

For the meat to be well digested, it must be eaten along with vegetable salads. Do not season them with mayonnaise, it should be discarded, but olive and sunflower oil should be included in the diet. Another condition is the rejection of simple carbohydrates. It is necessary to give preference to the so-called complex carbohydrates (vegetables, fruits, rye bread, cereals, and pasta from durum wheat). But cakes, soda, chips, chocolate, and other sweets will have to be excluded—no need to abandon them altogether.

Sometimes you can afford a little of those or other "harmful" products. Bans more than ever negatively affect the accumulation of excess weight in our body. Another group of products that reduce volume- These are foods rich in calcium, especially dairy. Calcium helps in burning fat, and almost 80% of fat is consumed from the abdomen. And of course, liquids. Drink more water, freshly squeezed fruit and vegetable juices, decoctions of herbs.

Exercises for the Abdomen

Exercises have a good effect on reducing the volume of the abdomen. Useful exercises for the press, cardio training, aerobics, and torsion hoop. Here are a few simple, but well-proven exercises that can restore your harmony and make your stomach flat. The main rule is the regularity and correctness of their implementation.

- Exercises Cat.
- Exercises Scissors.

- Air Energy Exercises.
- Exercises Tummy Tuck.
-

Exercises Cat

This is a beneficial exercise; it activates many muscle groups. Sit on your palms and knees, back and arms straight, look straight ahead. Bend your back, draw in your stomach as you exhale, relax, and take a deep breath. Hold your back in an arched position for 8-10 counts. Repeat exercise 10 times.

Exercises Scissors

This exercise allows you to strengthen muscles and remove fat in the abdomen. Lie on your back, straighten your legs. Put your hands under the buttocks, palms down. The main thing to monitor the lower back, it cannot be torn off the floor. Raise your legs 10-15 cm above the level. Make broad sweeps of your legs crosswise so that one leg is above the other (scissors). Socks are elongated. The exercise is performed on 8-10 counts. Breathe smoothly, exercise methodically, and vigorously. Do not lift your feet high and pull your socks.

Air Energy Exercises

This exercise is taken from Hatha Yoga. Everyone can do this exercise; he has no contraindications. Focus on your stomach and breath. Stand straight, feet shoulder-width apart, and arms lowered along the torso. Synchronously with sharp respiration through the nose, retract the stomach as far as you can. Then, on the contrary, with a sharp breath through the nose, push the stomach as far forward as possible. This exercise for the abdomen is performed at a fast pace, carefully monitors breathing and abdominal movements, they should be simultaneous. Repeat exercise 5 times. Increase the approaches gradually, bringing their number to 25.

Exercises Tummy Tuck

Another exercise from Hatha Yoga. It is done on holding your breath. The pose is the same as in the previous training. Exhale through the nose, while pausing; tilt the upper body by 45 degrees. Hands-on hips, fingers extended to the inguinal folds, stomach drawn to the spine. Focus on the area of the solar plexus, be in such a position as you can, holding your breath.

Then relax the abdominal muscles, take a shallow, shallow breath through the nose and return to the starting position. Perform the exercise once. Once you get used to it, having trained, it can be repeated two or three times, but no more. These exercises need to be supplemented with aerobic and cardio loads. Brisk walking, jogging, training on a stationary bike, a treadmill for half an hour a day will be enough. Dancing and aerobics are great.

Massage for the Abdomen

A massage is an excellent tool in the fight against excess fat. It improves metabolism, enhances blood circulation, and improves bowel function. Together, this helps to reduce the volume of the abdomen. The main rule is that you do not need to press hard and sincerely. The main methods of massage are rubbing and kneading the skin. Grab your abdomen with your fingers and knead it intensively with your fingertips. Grab the fold either horizontally or vertically concerning the chest. Vigorous rubbing spends clockwise, using the whole hand. Twitch and shake the fat folds intensively, pinch your skin. Firmly put your palms closed in the "castle" to the stomach from below, raising and lowering the stomach with short sharp movements. It is better to do this while sitting or standing. Massage should be done daily for 10 minutes. To increase the effect, use anti-cellulite creams, fat-burning oils.

Water Treatment

A douche with a contrast shower will help. Contrast shower helps to increase muscle tone, increase blood circulation, and improve the overall health of the body. You can also rub the skin on the stomach and sides with a hard washcloth in circular movements until red. The changes should be significant, but soft; the pressure should be superficial.

You can massage it with a steady stream of water from the shower, directing it in a circular motion to the abdomen. A bathhouse and a steam room with a broom help well. You can take special baths with oils of orange, lemon, peppermint, sea salt while gently massaging the skin of the abdomen underwater. The procedure lasts 20 minutes. The water should be warm. After a bath, rub yourself well with a hand towel.

Chapter 7

Mindset

So, do I think it's for everybody? Honestly, and no. I unquestionably don't accept that devouring throughout the day from 6 a.m. to 10 p.m. is for anyone. A couple of people may have to start with an increasingly delicate quick, et al. could undoubtedly bounce in with none weaning period with a 23 hour a day fasting window. Takeaway? Everybody is extraordinary. There is a comic that immediately shows a specialist recommending his patient beginning gradually by fasting between dinners. That might be an honest beginning.

My mentality has changed tons, within the last 3-4 years, as I even have perused, tuned in to people's accounts, and brought responsibility to possess wellbeing. So, here are a few of the items that I also have an inclination that I should note.

Manage Stress

If you are perpetually focused on, the pressure cycle must stop. At the purpose, once I was within the downright awful sleep deprivation, and at absolutely the bottom within the excursion, I had a 1-year-old, a multi-year-old, and a multi-year old – and that they were all reception since it had been summer. Within the fall, when my most established visited Kindergarten, and my center kid and younger youngster visited preschool two days hebdomadally, I had the choice to require a couple of to urge back some composure, commit once more to figure out, and despite the very fact that I hadn't changed much else, this had a considerable effect.

Perceive the stressors throughout your life. Be straightforward on the off chance that you need a break. And do not feel terrible that or engage contemplations that you "shouldn't" be focused otherwise; you "should" have the choice to affect it. Tell the "should beast" to go away. You're not God, you're human, and stress is awful for you. Whatever is causing it, I make some hard memories accepting that it might ever be justified, despite all the difficulty. You'll require an opportunity, and afterward, you'll continue your way of life once you feel stable. Or not. This prompts the subsequent idea.

Be Kind to Yourself

What I mean is, approve of the way that you are not great, should not be, and you're never going to be immediate. Adding to my pressure was the way that I feel I despised myself for not having the choice to try to all the items that I figured I "SHOULD" have the opportunity to decide to, the smallest amount of those things being to forego dessert or a glass of wine toward the day's end. Side note: I accept wound religious philosophy added to my issues since we expect that we need to have the choice to affect hard things with God's assistance. Or on the other hand, we need to have the opportunity to prevent negative behavior patterns with God's aid.

What's more, on the off chance that we will not affect hard things or stop negative behavior patterns, we expect that this is often because we aren't asking enough or perusing enough sacred writing or serving enough, which makes us increasingly miserable and discouraged. Stop the franticness – this is not the message of the Bible. A real ramification of the gospel message is this: RELAX. The KING has come, and he LOVES you, and zip on the earth can isolate you from him. On the off chance that your "gospel" is prompting will-love and self-humbling, at that time, you're not confiding within the original message of the Bible. On the off chance that you can't unwind in God's unlimited love for you, at that time, you'll always be unable to satisfy his motivation for you on the world. Try not to plan to do part B without section A.

Address Your Fears

Matt always wants to ridicule me since I might "choose" that I might accomplish something for a mind-blowing remainder. I might conclude I used to be never getting to eat dessert again. I might find that I used to be getting to awaken at 5:30 ordinarily to exercise for a vast remainder. It's practically humorous how frequently I even have done this type of thing to tumble off the wagon following seven days. These sorts of choices and this flawless attitude are 100% established in dread. Within the event that I can control my conduct, at that time, I can control my conditions and my life.

Holding firmly to control?? Look for the dread and manage it. At the purpose, once you can eliminate the fear in your life, you're opened to choose positive choices toward an objective, rather than attempting to accomplish the "objective" in one stage. On the off chance that model? Instead of going directly from a high-sugar, throughout the day eating way of life to a 20-hour quick, perhaps venture out moving breakfast back a few hours, or dinner up a few hours.

One final thing: Intermittent Fasting is an instrument, yet it is not the sole device. I think it's supernatural, as you almost certainly are aware. However, everybody is extraordinary; there could be something different happening in your body that may not happen in my body—thyroid, adrenal weakness, and so on. I frequently believe that since I had likewise gotten my gut and sugar yearnings leveled out a smidgen with supplements, that it genuinely pushed my change to IF. Smart dieting is an apparatus. Enhancements are an apparatus. Fasting may be a device.

There's not a one-size-fits-all methodology, and various people are sharing what has helped them. Will it help you? I trust during this way, yet on the off chance that it doesn't, it shouldn't cause despair. I even have attempted and bombed 1000 things. This one coincidentally worked on behalf of me, and that I found it at the right time when my body and my brain were prepared for it.

Additionally, despite the very fact that I feel serene and cheerful about where I'm, I'm an extended way from great and am continually learning and evolving. Probably the foremost enlightening people I tune as to if that's podcasters, creators, or my children's teachers admit to the way that they're Always attempting to enhance. Try not to pass judgment on your excursion!